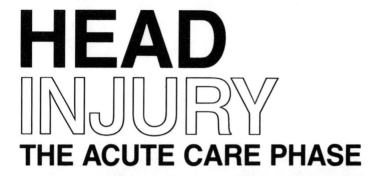

HEAD
INJURY
THE ACUTE CARE PHASE

Deborah Bidwell Manzi, BSN, CRRN
Patricia Allen Weaver, RPT

SLACK Incorporated, 6900 Grove Road, Thorofare, New Jersey 08086

Copyright © 1987 by SLACK Incorporated

Printed in the United States of America

Library of Congress Catalog Card Number: 86-4291

ISBN: 0-55642-001-3

Published by: SLACK Incorporated
               6900 Grove Rd.
               Thorofare, NJ 08086

Last digit is print number: 10   9   8   7   6   5   4   3   2   1

CONTENTS

PREFACE

As a certified rehabilitation nurse and admissions coordinator for a large head injury rehabilitation facility, I am often called upon to evaluate patients in the acute care setting and have thought "If only the staff had done this treatment, or tried that program, maybe we would have had a better chance to bring the patient to his fullest potential." This concern is what motivated Patricia Weaver (Director of Physical Therapy) and I to write the book.

As we researched the literature we found numerous articles on acute medical care of the head injured patient, diagnostic testing and long-term rehabilitation. Yet we found nothing which would help physical therapists working with the head injured patient in the acute care setting. This is what we have attempted to accomplish here.

This book is not intended to be the definitive text on head injury. It is meant to be a practical guide for the therapist working in the acute care setting who is treating head injured patients during the initial post-trauma period.

We hope that the therapists reading this book will take the information presented and enhance and expand on our ideas with their own in order to provide the most effective treatment possible.

Deborah Bidwell Manzi, BSN, CRRN
Patricia Allen Weaver, RPT

ACKNOWLEDGEMENTS

This book could never have been written without the help of many people. First, we are greatly indebted to Robert Sawicki, PhD, who authored the chapter on Functional Neuroanatomy and to James Mikula, PhD for his assistance and guidance in the initial planning of the text. A special thanks to Mr. Urban La Riccia, and to the administration and staff at Lake Erie Institute of Rehabilitation, without whose support and encouragement we may have given up. Special among these are Deborah Ferro, MA, CCC-SP/L, of the speech therapy department, for her contribution with the material on cognition, Debbie Kenny for her tireless efforts in editing and typing the manuscript, and Julie Posway and Willis Wright of the physical therapy department for their participation in the photographs.

On a day back in February 1986, as I sat in the Philadelphia airport waiting for my lost luggage (again), I met another traveler. We talked for a while about our jobs, and the usual exchange of business cards occurred. About a week or so later I received a call from that traveler asking me if I would consider submitting a proposal for a book on head injured patients. She asked that I include our Director of PT as co-author. After consulting with "Trish" and having several panic attacks, we decided to proceed. I would like to take a moment to thank that traveler, Judy Paquet, Acquisitions Editor, SLACK Incorporated for her faith in us, frequent pep talks, and sense of humor which kept us going.

Finally, and certainly not least, I would like to express our deepest appreciation to my husband Paul and to Trish's parents, Barbara and Maynard, for their love, support, and encouragement during the writing of this book.

Chapter 1

AN OVERVIEW

Head injury is a major cause of morbidity in the United States. According to statistics compiled by the National Head Injury Foundation, over 422,000 people sustain head injuries each year serious enough to be hospitalized.[1] Of these, approximately 25 percent (or 100,000) will require rehabilitation efforts after discharge from the acute care setting. Most will require a minimum of an interdisciplinary evaluation during the course of their acute hospital confinement.

The residual effects from a traumatic brain injury can run the gamut from mild memory problems to severe multimodality deficits, rendering the patient partially to totally dependent for all aspects of daily living skills. Head injured patients are different from other traumatically injured patients because of the cognitive and emotional problems they display. The therapist has to deal effectively with both the physical and cognitive rehabilitation of the patient. These must be carefully and effectively interfaced to allow the patient to reach his maximum potential.

Rehabilitation of the head injured patient cannot be deferred until he is transferred to a rehabilitation unit or facility. Ideally, it should begin in the intensive care unit. Many of the complications frequently seen in the head injured patient can be prevented or minimized with the establishment of an appropriate evaluation and treatment program while still in the acute care setting.

It is never too early to begin assessment and rehabilitation. A recent study by Weber[2] showed significant changes in EEG measurements with a noted cumulative effect in a group of patients who were started on a therapy regime three to six days post injury. In addition to EEG changes, increased alertness was noted in these patients, manifested by spontaneous eye opening, increased heart rate, and chewing motions. In addition, during continuous monitoring, a more normal sleep pattern was noted.[2] Cope and Hall[3] have also suggested earlier intervention of more active therapy procedures of auditory, proprioceptive, and tactile input to obtain active patient movement.

Jeannett and Bond,[4] during extensive studies, found that while recovery from closed head injury can continue for many years, the most rapid and spontaneous recovery generally occurs within the first year.

Since the head injured patient frequently sustains multiple trauma and numerous medical complications consistent with head injury, his stay in the acute care setting is often prolonged. It is not unusual for a rehabilitation facility to admit a patient several months post onset. Oftentimes, little if any rehabilitative efforts have been started. Frequently medical instability and use of a respirator are cited as the reasons.

In light of the previously mentioned studies, these reasons do not appear to be valid ones. Many secondary complications which can occur during a prolonged hospital stay can be prevented with the early institution of rehabilitation techniques. Pneumonia and respiratory complications can be prevented or minimized with chest physical therapy. This can be done even on the ventilator patient. Contractures can be prevented with range of motion programs which can be started as soon as orthopedic status is determined to rule out fractures. Spasticity and formation of heterotopic ossification can be prevented with administration of appropriate relaxation techniques and medications. Intensive multimodality stimulation can be performed to prevent the sensory deprivation often seen in patients with prolonged stays in the intensive care unit.

The physical therapist can and should play an important role in the initiation of these techniques. Often as the only therapist on staff in a small hospital, with her knowledge of neurophysiology, she can be the prime motivator of therapeutic intervention.

What has been attempted in this text is to give the therapist the theoretical framework and practical ideas to be able to effect a program of rehabilitation techniques which can be initiated for the head injured patient within a day or two of admission to the acute care facility.

References

1. Anderson DW, McLaurin RL (Eds): Report on national head and spinal cord survey, conducted for the National Institute of Neurological and Communicative Disorders and Stroke. J Neurosurg 1980;(suppl)(November):S1-S43.
2. Weber PL: Sensorimotor therapy: Its effects on EEG's of acute comatose patients. Arch Phys Med Rehabil 1984;65:45-47.
3. Cope DN, Hall K: Head injury rehabilitation: Benefit of early intervention. Arch Phys Med Rehabil 1982;63:433.
4. Jeannett B, Bond M: Assessment of outcome after severe brain damage. Lancet 1975;1:480.

Chapter 2

Robert Sawicki, PhD

FUNCTIONAL NEUROANATOMY

The traditional approach to the description of the brain's interconnections follows a model of "the-shinbone's-connected-to-the-ankle-bone," with relative disregard for the functions which are subserved by the various connections and interconnections. In a monograph such as this, the intent of which is to provide a description of methods which may be applied to the assessment of traumatically brain injured persons, such a model does not suffice. Instead, one must start from the premise that the brain is the central organ of information processing, and that the brain is the organ which mediates the majority of response innervation. Thus the various landmarks, lobes, and strata must be placed in the context of the functions which they appear to facilitate. The purpose of this chapter is to provide such a context, to the extent known, in relation to brain structure. In order to provide some working assumptions for brain-behavior relations, a model of functional interaction with physiology will also be reviewed.

Basic Physiology

The average human brain weighs approximately 1450 g, with the average brain weight for females being approximately 10 percent less. The latter difference appears to be related to height and overall body weight.[1] In terms of volume, this suggests a range of 1000 cc to 2000 cc.[2] Though the brain accounts for only approximately ⅟₅₀ of total body weight, it requires nearly one fifth of cardiac output (at rest) to maintain necessary levels of oxygen and glucose.[3] Because the brain is unable to independently manufacture energy sources, neural metabolism notably changes after 6 seconds of cerebrovascular interruption; after two minutes of such interruption affected brain activity stops; and after five minutes, infarction begins.[3] The brain requires such high energy levels to maintain its role in information processing, body and environmental monitoring, conscious responding, and autonomic functioning.

The brain sits in the cranial cavity bathed and cushioned by cerebrospinal fluid. Both the brain and spinal cord are covered by three layers of protective tissue, the meninges. The outside covering, the dura mater, is relatively thick and relatively hard, suggesting the consistency of gelatinous, high quality writing paper. The next layer toward the brain is the arachnoid, which has a weblike appearance and follows the overall contours of the brain. The final layer, the pia, intimately adheres to the contours of the nervous system, and on initial inspection is difficult to discriminate from the cortex itself.

Nutrients and oxygen are brought to the brain by means of the two internal carotid arteries (anteriorally) and the two vertebral arteries posteriorally. The brain itself is irrigated by three major sets of arteries: the anterior cerebral and middle cerebral, which are primarily fed by the internal carotid arteries, and the posterior cerebral arteries, which branch from the basilar artery. The basilar artery forms on the underside (ventral portion) of the brain stem, at the level of the pons, from the juncture of the two vertebral arteries. This system is highly interconnected (anastomosis), thus allowing compensatory flow for substantial levels of blockage. The remainder of arterial irrigation is provided by branches from these major vessels. It is of interest to note that the majority of strokes occur in the left, middle cerebral artery or its tributaries. Such stroke produced the often observed syndrome of right hemiplegia and aphasia (language disturbance).

The Neuron

The *neuron* is the basic unit of the brain and the basic mechanism for information processing. The neuron is a cell composed of soma or cell body, an axon, and dendrites. The soma contains the nucleus of the cell. The axon extends from the soma. Though each neuron only contains a single axon, an axon may have multiple branches. At the end of the axon are terminal boutons intended for connection with other neurons. Information which has moved along the axon will pass to other cells through these terminals (telodentria). Dendrites are the structures by which a neuron receives information from other cells. They increase the likelihood of a cell's being activated, since they increase the surface area available for stimulation. Axon terminals interface with dendrites. This area of interface is called a synapse.

Though the synapse is not a structure but the contact space between cells, it is very important for information transmission. It is through this space (synaptic cleft) that neurotransmitters flow to transmit the nerve impulse to additional neurons. Synapses may be of various types: axon terminal-dendrite (axodendritic), terminal-terminal (axosynaptic), terminal-soma (axosomatic), terminal-axon (axoaxonic), dendrite-dendrite (dendrodendritic). Synapses directly to the cell body are presumed to be more influential to cell response than more peripheral contacts.[2]

Types of Neurons

There are three general types of neurons. *Unipolar* cells have only an axon and are usually found in the spinal ganglia and portions of the trigeminal nerve. The *bipolar* cells mediate sensory information. Descriptively, bipolar cells are characterized by one main dendrite and on the other side of the cell body a single axis cylinder. *Multipolar* neurons are the most prevalent cells. They mediate both sensory and motor information. Multipolar cells may be found throughout the central and autonomic systems. Descriptively, they are characterized by flourishing dendritic patterns such as the heavily forested Purkinje's cells of the cerebellum.

Additionally, neurons have also been classified by their size. Those sending axons for long distances have been classified as Golgi Type I (e.g., peripheral motor neurons), while neurons with short axons have been classified as Golgi Type II (e.g., associated neurons).

Sensory neurons may be classified into three general types. The *exteroceptors* receive information from the body surface and respond to tactual sensation, thermal changes, visual or auditory displays, olfactory stimuli, and pain. *Proprioceptors* mediate kinesthetic awareness. They transmit information from joints, capsules, ligaments, and fascia. *Interoceptors* receive input from primarily autonomic areas; that is, they grossly mediate information regarding gastrointestinal processes, respiratory efficiency, hydration, nutritional status, and sexual responsiveness.

Nerve Impulse or Signal

Actual signal transmission along a neuron has both chemical and electrical properties. Chemically, once stimulated, the cell membrane of a neuron undergoes a reaction (depolarization) which alters its permeability to sodium (Na^+) and potassium (K^+). This is the action potential, which, once stimulated, produces the nerve impulse. As Na^+ passes into the cell and K^+ moves out through the cell wall at successive points (sodium-potassium pump) the signal moves along the axon toward the terminals. The passage of this nerve impulse may be measured electrically. It is this activity from which electroencephalogram (EEG) readings are taken.

Since the action potential is regarded as an "all-or-none" phenomenon, intensity of response is related to frequency of cell firing and the recruitment of additional neurons rather than individual signal strength. Efficiency of signal transmission is related to two factors. The first is caliber, or thickness of the axon. Thicker axons allow faster signal transmission. The presence of myelin is the other factor. As myelin (a glial cell) wraps around the axon, clefts are produced between glial cells. The nerve impulse jumps between these clefts (nodes of Ranvier), thus moving more quickly than if it were only along the immediate length of an axon. This process is called *saltatory conduction*. Myelin serves the additional function of insulating individual nerve fibers and preventing the impulse from dispersing before it reaches target structures. The effects of demyelination can readily be seen in disorders like the Guillain-Barré syndrome.

Effects of Cell Injury

Though the common analogy for a neuron is a telephone wire, the neuron is a cell. Thus its overall composition is that of an aqueous structure surrounded by a membrane. Nutrients are transported through the length of this structure and waste is removed. Destruction of the membrane or transection of the cell causes this process to cease. The following is a summary of events after experimental transection of an axon: the axon and myelin in the vicinity of the injury rapidly degenerate. In the brain and spinal cord, a glial scar quickly forms in and around the area of injury. According to Kelly's[4] description, after two to three days, effects of the injury are seen in the cell body. If the soma does not survive, degeneration proceeds outward and destroys the remainder of the axon proximal to the injury. Initial effects may be noted in the axon terminals, distal to the injury, at approximately one day after the injury. *Terminal degeneration* occurs in about two weeks.

Over the following two to three months, the axon distal to the injury degenerates (wallerian degeneration). Though not directly affected by the lesion, neurons dependent on the transected neuron for stimulation may secondarily degenerate due to loss of stimulation (transneuronal degeneration), thus starting the process over again. Review of the time periods involved in such degeneration, and the possibility that terminals which may be junctures for other cells may take several weeks to die, suggest reasons for functional losses which may develop at some distance to the actual traumatic brain injury.

Injured cells attempt to regenerate through a process involving *chromatolysis*, that is, a dissolution and later reorganization of nuclear material. The process necessitates major protein synthesis and lasts several weeks. Subsequently to re-establishing the cell body, the neuron attempts to re-establish terminal connections. Of note is the finding that chromatolysis is insufficient to insure cell survival, since viable connections must be regained to prevent atrophy, which leads to reinitiating the process of degeneration. This seems to be the underlying phenomenon which comprises the functional regeneration of central neural tissue. Additionally, some cells degenerate so quickly that the process is not given opportunity to start (e.g., thalamic neurons).[4]

Functional Systems

Conventionally, when describing neural organization, one refers to the various areas of the brain, which have been named after the bones of the skull that lie above that brain area (e.g., frontal, parietal, temporal, occipital). However, in keeping with the intent of this chapter, brain organization will be described in terms of functional involvement rather than solely in terms of cranial geography. This approach to describing the interaction of neural substrates with behavior is exemplified by the work of A.R. Luria.[5]

Luria's model may be described as a compromise between the view that behavioral functions are strictly represented in discrete parts of the brain (localizationalist theory) and the view that the total brain is involved in all activity (equipotentialist theory). Luria's model is based on the concept of the functional system. Brain organization is considered to be dynamic in terms of involving brain mediated processes to the extent that they are necessary for a given act or mental formulation. Thus, though written composition varies from oral reading in that one necessitates manual output while the other demands speech, both performances demand access to a lexicon, and both demand controlled sequential movement. Thus, while the neuron is the basic unit of information processing, the functional system is the relative unit of neural to behavioral translation.

Luria[6] provides a physical example to indicate how functional systems can also come into play when an organism attempts to accommodate to injury:

> . . . *if the principal group of muscles working during respiration (the diaphragm) ceases to act, the intercostal muscles are brought into play, but if for some reason or other they are impaired, the muscles of the larynx are mobilized and the animal or person begins to swallow air, which thus reaches the alveoli of the lungs by a completely different route.*

Similarly, if the neural area mediating vocal labeling (naming) is compromised, an individual attempts to communicate the intended label by describing the object by its characteristics or functions. Thus, communication is achieved by an alternate route. The functional system therefore is a complex interaction between relatively simple, primary brain functions, complex associative functions, and hypercomplex executive brain functions which are responsible for ongoing accuracy monitoring, revision, and planning. Thus, Luria postulated three basic functional units for the brain: (a) functions involved in the regulation of overall cortical tone or arousal; (b) functions involved in receiving information from the outside world, processing it, and storing it; and (c) functions involved in organizing activity, planning activity, verifying activity, and reviewing/verifying overall mental processes. As one can read, these functions are notably interdependent. Sufficient arousal must be activated for sensation to be recorded and processed; and both optimal arousal and accurate sensation must occur for activity to be accurate and useful. Moving in the opposite direction, accurate monitoring must occur to place incoming information into the appropriate contexts, adjust arousal, and so forth.

Applying Luria's model, the brain areas most involved in arousal appear to lie in the midbrain and brain stem. These have been grouped under the title of the *reticular activating system*. Rather than following a diagram, you may use your own head to localize the primary sensory areas. The primary area for vision lies at the back of the brain (occipital area), thus it is at the back of your head, above where the neck muscles insert into the back of the skull. The primary area for hearing lies at the sides of the brain (temporal area); thus, on your head this area is approximately just above and behind where your ears are. If you draw a line from the top front of one ear to the top front of the other ear, the area in front of that line (frontal area) approximates the position of the primary motor area, and the region behind the line (parietal area) approximates the position of the primary somatosensory area. The primary area for smell is on the underside of the brain, above and behind the eyes.

The primary areas occupy a relatively small volume in the lobe or brain area which they occupy. Near to, and usually surrounding each primary sensory area is a secondary area. Unlike the primary area which appears to respond to the presence of a particular stimuli, secondary areas are presumed to respond to the pattern in which the stimuli occur. Surrounding the secondary are tertiary, or associative areas which facilitate the interaction among sensory areas. Thus, a viewed object may also have a sound (word/name) associated with it. Or, one may read a word (visual input) and associate the conceptual meaning of that word, which may also include a mental-tactual sensation (e.g., "silk stockings"). Memories are the most complex example of such tertiary interaction among sensory areas. Tertiary areas also permit the interaction of sensation with motor response (e.g., writing to dictation, constructing an object from a blueprint).

In addition to facilitating motor movement, the frontal lobes, which lie in the front of that imaginary line, facilitate the complex activities of initiating, monitoring, revising, and planning, as well as reviewing mental activity on the whole. From this review of the interaction among functional units, one may begin to get a sense of the pattern of neuronal interconnections within the brain. Obviously, the interconnection from the frontal areas to the rest of the brain will be the richest. It is the quantity of these cortico-cortical connections (the neocortex), which anatomically differentiates the human brain from the brain of other neighboring species. It is suggested that these connections are the substrate which allows human beings to imagine, as well as to act. In the next section, a more traditional review of the major brain areas, their usual connections, and presumed function is offered.

The Reticular Activating System: Arousal

Below the cerebral hemispheres and in front of (anterior) to the cerebellar hemispheres, lies a stalk of neural tracts which extend upward to the midbrain (i.e., the upper end of the stalk and surrounding tissue, located in the midline, below the level of the hypothalamus; chief structures are the tectum, tegmentum, and the cerebral aqueduct), and downward, past the pons and the fourth ventricle, to the spinal column. This stalk is the medulla oblongata. Within this system is a set of highly interconnected, intermingled neurons with multiple connections in the cerebral hemispheres, basal ganglia, cerebellum, and spinal cord. The major function appears to be one of interrelating and organizing various sensory information (interoceptive, proprioceptive, and exteroceptive) to facilitate the preparation for a response appropriate to the situation. In addition, the reticular system appears to play a role in maintaining and adjusting arousal, regulating degree of muscle tone, facilitating the somatic and autonomic motor responses necessary for respiration, as well as vasomotor responses and cardiac responses.[7]

Based on animal studies, injuries in portions of the reticular system affect sleep/wake patterns. Substantial midbrain lesions which affect reticular tracts produce coma. Interruption of reticular-cortical connections interfere with preparatory arousal (alerting/orienting responses) necessary for efficient responsiveness. The cortex and reticular system appear to have reciprocal interactions; that is, in addition to being stimulated by the reticular system, the cortex sends back feedback which can then alter the arousal potential of certain kinds of information (i.e., psychological meaning).[8]

Thus, the reticular system plays both a major facilitating role and modulating role in promoting adaptive responsiveness throughout the brain. Though one may quickly see that an injury to the reticular system may directly affect arousal, given the interactive component, one must also recognize that an injury to a cortical area which provides feedback will also affect arousal for certain kinds of information indirectly.

The Cerebellum: Integration, Coordination, and Adjustment

When quickly viewed, the two cerebellar hemispheres appear as miniatures of the two cerebral hemispheres which lie above them. The cerebellar tonsils lie beneath the occipital area and are connected to the brain stem at the level of the fourth ventricle. The cerebellum receives information which deals with muscle activity in terms of stretch and joint activity. It also receives postural information and monitors equilibrium through vestibular connections. The cerebellum also plays an integrating role in spinal and cranial movement. There is also a suggestion that the cerebellum plays a role in initiating learned motor responses.[7]

Injuries to the cerebellum often produce *asynergia* or ataxia (defective integration and modulation of agonists, antagonists, and fixators), *dysmetria* (difficulty gauging movement orientation and extension), *dysdiadochokinesis* (breakdown in unilaterally, rapidly alternating movements), *intention tremor* (uncontrolled oscillation in a limb during a voluntary movement which appears to increase as the goal is approximated), and *rebound effects* (inability to control/modulate/terminate the extent of a movement). Visual-motor symptoms (nystagmus) and vocal-motor symptoms (dysarthria) may also be seen, as well as what appear to be balance disturbances.

The Basal Ganglia: Supplementary Motor Facilitation

The basal ganglia are several subcortical neural areas that appear to produce effects on the speed and volitional control of motor movement. The basal ganglia are located in the internal, middle section of the brain below and lateral to the thalamus. This area is usually defined by the following structures; caudate nucleus, putamen, globus pallidus, and the amygdala. These structures have also been identified as the extrapyramidal motor system. Though this area has not been defined in terms of primary motor function, it plays a facilitory role in motor movement. Injuries to this system produce changes in the speed of muscular movement (e.g., changes in facial expressions, blinking, and total gait rhythm). Overall disturbance is thought to be secondary to increased muscular tone which then limits the fine postural adjustments which accompany global, voluntary movements. Spasticity is a common concomitant of injury to this area. When cortical control of this area is compromised, involuntary movement patterns may appear (e.g., dystonia, choreiform movements, hemiballismus, athetosis).

The Thalamus and Hypothalamus

The thalamus is a major relay station for sensory and motor information between complex cerebral areas and subcortical facilitory areas. Because of its multiple connections and its integrative position among various sensory tract connections, a role in attentional shifting has been postulated for the thalamus.[9] Thalamic-reticular connections support notions of such a role. Though losses in many complex reasoning activities are usually attributed to cortical lesions, disruption of the thalamus also produces many of these same symptoms (e.g., left thalamic lesions tend to produce aphasic-type disturbances, while right thalamic lesions affect perceptual-spatial performance). Emotional apathy and irritability have both been noted after thalamic injuries, though at varying thalamic sites. Such findings do not suggest redundancy between cortical and thalamic function; however, they may be understood as the effect of destruction of a traffic control center on the flow of information through that center.

The hypothalamus is primarily involved in autonomic functioning. In addition to direct facilitation of functions involving hunger and thirst, body temperature, and sleep cycles, the hypothalamus also exerts indirect control of bodily functions, arousal, and emotional reactivity through hormonal stimulation. Thus, injury to the hypothalamus may present with symptoms as varied as sleep disturbance to hyperthermia to sexual impotence to diabetes insipidus.

The Limbic System: Emotional Reactivity

Though many of its structures overlap with structures included in other "definitional" brain regions, the limbic area has been defined as a functionally interrelated neural system. The components of the system usually include the pre-optic area, the hypothalamus, the anterior thalamus, a portion of the upper middle thalamus, the epithalamus, the amygdaloid system, the septum, upper midbrain, and cortical components including the hippocampus, olfactory areas, cingulate, and sub-callosum. The neural strata in the system appear to be a transition between "old brain" and neocortex. As may be understood from the structures included, the limbic area is readily involved in sensory integration and arousal. However, unlike prior areas mentioned, connections to the hypothalamus and amygdaloid circuits allow emotional texture to be added to the information being processed. Given the connections to hippocampal areas which are involved in the transmission of information to storage, a partial role for the limbic system is one of emotionally tagging information to help discriminate the relative importance of a piece of information. Autonomic connections are involved in generating physiological preparatory states for either self-defense or avoidance. The overall reactivity of limbic arousal and activating centers appear to be under cortical inhibitory and modulatory control.

Thus, limbic lesions which result in emotional dyscontrol and hyper-reactivity may more likely indicate disconnection from cortical inhibitory centers than direct limbic lesion effect.

Cerebral Asymmetry and Functional Lateralization

Though the overall appearance of the cerebral hemispheres is of two symmetrical lobes, anatomically there are minor differences. The following summary of asymmetries is taken from a review by Kolb and Whishaw[2]:

1. Differences in the specific gravity of the two hemispheres suggest that the left hemisphere has more grey matter (neuronal muscle) than the right.

2. The temporal lobes demonstrate a notable asymmetry, which first appears in the last fetal trimester. It is characterized by a larger planum temporale on the left and a more sizable area for primary auditory cortex (Heschl's gyrus) on the right. The differences are presumed to be the anatomical basis for language (left temporal) and musical functions (right temporal). A complimentary asymmetry is evident in the thalamus.

3. The temporo-parietal cortex lying below the sylvian fissure (upper border of the temporal lobe) appears larger on the right. This difference is presumed to be related to the greater specialization of right hemisphere for spatial integration of sensory information.

4. Broca's area on the left shows greater sulcal invagination (fissure depth), while the similar area on the right exposes greater surface cortex (gyral area). Again, the difference suggests an anatomical substrate for language.

5. Grossly, the left hemisphere extends further occipitally, while the right extends further frontally. In contrast, the posterior horns of the lateral ventricles are more likely to extend further on the right.

6. There is a relationship between some hemispheric asymmetries and gender and handedness.

In terms of specific functional systems, the following asymmetries may be noted:

1. Visual fields, not ocular connections, are represented in the contralateral hemisphere; for example, information from the left visual field is processed in the right posterior area. Each eye, however, sends information to

both hemispheres. The nasal eye-field sends information to the ipsalateral hemisphere, while the peripheral field sends information to the contralateral hemisphere.

2. Auditorially, though the system does not appear to be significantly as crossed as vision (the greater redundancy appears to be related to the abilities related to sound localization), information from the right ear appears to show greater activation in the left hemisphere, and vice versa.

3. Motorically and sensorially, the information processing system appears almost completely crossed.

4. In terms of preferential processing of information, to relative degrees, language-related information (especially words) and language-related gestures tend to show greater activation in the left hemisphere. In contrast, nonspeech sounds, melodies, spatial information, and information requiring nonverbal multisensory integration show greater right hemisphere activation. Pattern recognition through various sensory modalities appears to have greater right hemisphere activation, which also suggests a role for the right hemisphere in spatially patterned movement.

Geographic Divisions of the Cortex

The Frontal Areas

Geographically, the frontal lobes constitute all of the brain areas anterior to the central sulcus. The frontal cortex is richly, for the most part reciprocally, connected with most of the remainder of cortical and subcortical areas. It receives input from the somatosensory, auditory, and visual areas in relays through the parietal areas. Subcortically, the frontal cortex receives information from limbic structures (caudate, hypothalamus, amygdaloid system), the thalamus, and the basal ganglia. It also receives information from the cerebellum and the spinal cord. Information is returned to many of these same structures. In terms of important areas for functional processing, there are rich connections to the association areas within the temporal and parietal cortex.

As stated earlier in this chapter, and as may be understood from its pattern of interconnections, the frontal cortex is intimately involved in monitoring, reviewing, revising, and planning. Given the effects of injuries in the frontal areas, it is also involved in both initiating and terminating behavioral responses, as well as modulating social and sexual responsiveness. For a complete review of frontal cortical functioning, the reader is referred to Stuss and Benson.[10]

The functional involvement of the frontal lobes may be defined in terms of several classes of performance, which are disturbed after injury to that area.

1. **Controlled motor movement**. In addition to *apraxia* which is defined as the "impairment of ability to carry purposeful movements by the individual who has normal primary motor skills (strength, reflexes, coordination) and normal comprehension of the act to be carried out . . .,"[11] disorders affecting the ability to initiate planned movements are evident. Motor programs disintegrate into stereotyped components, which may be perseveratively repeated. Verbal control over performance may be disconnected. Thus, responses may not be inhibited on demand. Inaccurate comparisons are likely to occur between targeted and actual performance. More frustrating to the individual, differences may appear between intended and actual movements.

2. **Attention**. This process may be defined as the capacity to direct mental processes and to purposefully exercise selectivity in terms of both screening one set of inputs over another and selecting one set of responses over another.

3. **Awareness**. When disturbed, this process demonstrates the gamut of symptoms from inattention to specific bodily parts (e.g., denial of a limb), to blunted affect or frank apathy to denial of disability. The underlying disturbance is not perceptual per se, but appears to be a disconnection from the meaning of what is observed or a disturbance of affectively mediated motor adjustment.

4. **Personality and emotional control**. Changes appear related to difficulties in modulating emotional reactivity, exaggeration of previously socialized (inhibited) personality characteristics, and overall irritability. Self-reports by traumatically brain injured persons indicate that a component of the ongoing interpersonal irritability is a lack of ability to maintain a predictive attitude in social contexts; that is, social cues are misread and the subtleties of nonverbal communication are lost, thus the individual becomes purely reactive instead of participatory. Thus, the social situation becomes least tolerable because of the ongoing demands for rapid conceptual comprehension and continuous, subtle performance adjustments.

5. **Language**. Both the regulatory power of language and the fluency of language may be compromised. Frontal disturbance appears to limit both the ability to organize spoken communication and to organize the comprehension of demands which require multi-step performance. Primarily frontal disturbance plays a role in language disturbances characterized by limitations of oral verbal output.

6. **Memory**. The frontal cortex appears to play a role in organizing information and maintaining the discreteness of stored sets of information. Frontal areas also play a role in knowing that something has been stored

and whether what is recalled approximates the stored information. Thus, confabulation is more likely with anterior brain dysfunction.

The Temporal Cortex

The temporal areas are a pair of peninsulas which lie laterally below the frontal areas, with the posterior temporal areas lying below the parietal areas, and anterior to the occipital areas. They are the location of the primary auditory and secondary auditory cortex. Kolb and Whishaw[2] postulate three general functions for the temporal areas: processing auditory sensation, as well as auditory and visual perceptual processing; special transfer capability for long-term information storage; and the coloring of sensory information with affective tone. Based on prior descriptions of functional areas, one may readily postulate the expected connections for temporal areas (e.g., input [afferent] connections from primary sensory areas, out [efferent] connections to the limbic system and frontal association areas). Temporal areas have been reported as especially sensitive to irritative lesions, thus they are prominent in seizure disorders. A review of disturbances after temporal injury will provide some insight into the mediating functions of the temporal cortex.

1. **Sensory selectivity**. Disturbance in the temporal area appears to produce inattention to sensations which are typically processed by that area (e.g., verbal information on the left, tonal/melodic information on the right). Thus on recall, information appears to be lost because it was ignored rather than misperceived. Visual information is affected similarly, based on visual field representation; however, lesions in the right temporal area appear to create bilateral effects.[2]
2. **Visual perception**. Complex pattern processing and comprehension, whether the information be faces or nonverbal social cues, appear to be affected.
3. **Language**. Comprehension disorders are classically associated with posterior left temporal lesions. Clinically, hyperfluency has also been reported with temporal lesions.
4. **Memory**. Associations between memory disturbance and temporal disturbance have been consistently noted, with the hippocampal regions playing a central role in memory processing. The function appears to be one of transmission rather than actual storage, since disturbance is noted in recent events and in learning after the lesion rather than in long-term recall.
5. **Personality**. Changes associated with temporal disturbance include preoccupation with relatively minor details, perseverative discussions of personal problems without regard to the context in which they are being

discussed, religious preoccupation, and a tendency toward aggressive acting out. Indiscriminate hypersexuality has also been reported.

The Parietal Cortex

The parietal areas are located behind the central fissure, above the temporal areas, and in front of the occipital areas. The parietal cortex appears to have two major roles: one of mediating sensory and perceptual information gathered throughout the body, and the other of integrating the sensory input from the primary sensory regions (auditory, visual, somatic, etc.). In addition to inputs from primary and secondary areas, the parietal cortex receives input from the thalamus and hypothalamus. Thalamic connections are reciprocal. It also sends information to portions of the basal ganglia, midbrain, and spinal cord, as well as the association areas of the frontal and temporal cortices.

From earlier discussions of Luria's model of brain-behavior relationships, one may readily infer that parietal cortex is a tertiary functional area; that is, it is multisensory integrative. Its motor and sensory role will be discussed separately.

Parietal motor integration appears to be related to motor functioning in a three-dimensional space. The effect is one of providing information for controlled muscular orientation rather than primary muscular innervation. Thus, limb apraxia may also be seen secondary to parietal lesions.

A review of the effects of parietal disturbance will provide further examples of parietal functioning.

1. **Academic skills**. Lesions in the left parietal area have been notably involved in arithmetic disturbance (acalculia), reading disabilities (alexia), and writing disturbance (agraphia). Right/left confusion has also been associated with left parietal dysfunction. In terms of academic skills, an underlying compromise of symbol translation appears to be a consistent contributory factor.
2. **Memory**. Disturbances in short-term delayed recall are evident.
3. **Spatial disturbance**. The overall description of parietal involvement in mental spatial representation appears to be limited by our ability to verbally describe these essentially nonverbal functions. However, three general types of disturbances are notable: those having to do with bodily representation (e.g., body image distortion, right/left confusion, neglect syndromes); disturbances having to do with spatial perception (e.g., topographical orientation, angular recognition); and spatial-motor disturbance (e.g., constructional apraxia, dressing apraxia).
4. **Disconnection syndromes**. Various agnosias (visual or tactual) which limit the recognition of objects in various sensory modalities. These are

not naming disorders, but a lack of comprehension for the object perceived.

5. **Tactual disorders**. Dysfunctions characterized by inaccurate tactual localization, as well as misperceptions during complex tactual discriminations.

The Occipital Cortex

Located in the posterior cerebrum, the occipital cortex contains the primary and secondary visual areas. Though complex in their handling of visual information, the occipital areas demonstrate a relatively simpler organization of input and output in comparison to the other cerebral areas. The organization of the occipital cortex is more modality specific than other brain areas.

Areas of Sensitivity to Traumatic Brain Injury

Though the overall focus here has been on brain functions, and the effects of lesions have been used to support assumptions of local involvement, it is also necessary to introduce the general effects of traumatic injury on the brain. Because of its situation within the cranium and because of the fragile connections created by the midbrain and brain stem, several brain areas are consistently more susceptible to traumatic disruption than others. Injuries which produce gyratory (twisting) force on the brain disturb white matter (myelinated axons) connections within the brain. Thus major effects are noted among associative functions. In addition, brainstem strain produces effects in the reticular system, thus creating effects which range from unconsciousness/coma to momentary disorientation.

Because of their location behind the cranial orbits, the temporal and orbital frontal areas are in a unique position to be consistently bruised. Thus, memory disturbance becomes a relatively constant concomitant of even minor head injury, with the degree of hippocampal injury reflecting the degree of memory disturbance. In addition, at least mild fluctuations in attention and personality are likely secondary to the frontal involvement.

Parietal areas are susceptible to both direct and contre-coup effects because of their geographic location. Due to the presence of watershed arterial irrigation, they are also susceptible to secondary hypoxic effects.

Summary

As we have proceeded through this summary of functional neuroanatomy, it has hopefully become obvious that brain functioning is dynamic. In subtle and complex ways, each component of the brain plays a role in adaptive human activity, and that role varies, depending on the system demands of the given activity. Thus, there really are no "silent" areas of the brain, and given its overall organization, it would be difficult to demonstrate that one area takes over the functions of another area after an injury. Instead, subtle variation in dynamic involvement likely occurs, which permits the goals of an activity to be accomplished in different but adaptive ways.

References

1. Duchen LW: General pathology of neurons and neurologia. In Adams JH, Corsekis JAN, Duchen LW (Eds): Greenfield's Neuropathology. Ed 4. John Wiley and Sons Inc, New York, 1984.
2. Kolb B, Whishaw IA: Fundamentals of Human Neuropsychology. WH Freeman, New York, 1985.
3. Hachinski V, Naris JW: The Acute Stroke. FA Davis Publishers, Philadelphia, 1985.
4. Kelly JP: Reaction of neurons to injury. In Kandel ER, Schwarts JH (Eds): Principles of Neural Science. Elsevier/North-Holland, New York, 1981.
5. Luria AR: Higher Cortical Functions in Man. Basic Books Inc, New York, 1980.
6. Luria AR: The Working Brain: An Introduction to Neuropsychology. Basic Books Inc, New York, 1973.
7. Peele TL: The Neuroanatomic Basis for Clinical Neurology. McGraw-Hill Publishers, New York, 1977.
8. Plum F, Posner JB: The Diagnosis of Stupor and Coma. FA Davis Publishers, Philadelphia, 1983.
9. McGhie A: Psychological aspects of attention and its disorders. In Vinken PJ, Gruyn GW (Eds): Handbook of Clinical Neurology. Vol 3. John Wiley & Sons Inc, New York, 1969.
10. Stuss DT, Benson DF: The Frontal Lobes. Raven Press Publishers. New York, 1986.
11. Hecaen H: Apraxia. In Filskov SB, Ball TJ (Eds): Handbook of Clinical Neuropsychology. John Wiley & Sons Inc, New York, 1981.

Chapter 3

COMPLICATIONS OF HEAD INJURY

One of the reasons that treating the head injured patient is so challenging to the therapist and other members of the treatment team is that no two head injured patients are ever alike. While the medical complications are vast enough, ranging from multiple secondary brain insults (from later developing hematomas, for example) to cardiovascular and respiratory problems, the head injured patient may often have many other complications with which the therapist may not be familiar.

Whereas the patient who suffers a cardiovascular accident tends to have a very focal injury, which often will respond to a specific neurophysiological treatment, the head injured patient usually suffers highly diffuse damage. Not only does this cause the neurophysiological problems of the stroke patient, but it also creates additional complications of memory and perceptual disorders, along with potential behavioral and psychosocial problems.

In this chapter on complications of head injury, we have focused on what we believe to be the most frequently seen complications from medical, cognitive, neuromotor, and behavioral aspects and their specific relationship to the head injury patient in the acute care setting.

Medical Complications

Coma

Coma is considered to be a prolonged and profound loss of consciousness in which a patient may show no reaction to painful stimuli, or may react with a primative defense movement such as limb withdrawal.[1] The initial period of coma is believed to be due to widespread damage to white matter which is associated with disconnection of large areas of the cerebral cortex from subcortical structures.[2] Deepening coma is usually associated with cerebral contusions, lacerations, and hematomas which can lead to increased intracranial pressure and brain shift.

Length of coma is often used as a factor in determining severity of injury, and as a prognostic indicator of recovery. It is widely accepted that Jeannett and Teasdale[3] have made the greatest strides in understanding coma and predicting outcome of injury.

The longer the suppression of conscious function, the more serious the injury.[4] While in coma, the patient is unable to function at any conscious level. He has no volitional control over any bodily function and all activities of daily living must be performed for him.

The true period of coma is actually short-lived. The EEG of a patient in coma will show a continuous sleeplike pattern.[5] Continuous sleeplike coma almost never lasts more than two to four weeks.

Beyond a period of about four weeks, the patient passes into what is known as a persistent vegetative state. This is described as a state in which the patient remains unresponsive. He often appears awake at times, and exhibits only vegetative functions, such as spontaneous respirations, excretory functions, and perhaps swallowing. The patient in a persistent vegetative state, however, will have EEG patterns demonstrating definite sleep/wake cycles.[5]

The most frequently used measure of the severity of brain injury is the Glasgow Coma Scale, which will be discussed in detail in Chapter 4.

Respiratory Problems

Respiratory problems are one of the most frequent complications of severe traumatic brain injury. They may be primary, such as a pneumothorax; a blocked airway, which may occur at the time of injury; or depressed respiratory function, which can occur at any time during the acute stabilization period. The latter is often caused by increased intracranial pressure. Secondary causes of respiratory difficulty include brainstem injury, bilateral hemispheric dysfunction, subarachnoid hemorrhage, or extrinsic factors such as pulmonary edema.

If coughing reflexes are depressed or absent, the patient will need to be closely monitored in order to maintain oxygenation and prevent aspiration. An excess of secretions is often found in the head injured patient from both the air passages and the salivary glands. Chest physical therapy is often very effective in clearing the lungs of the patient with an inadequate cough.

Maintenance of adequate oxygenation may require intubation, mechanical ventilation, or tracheostomy. Clinical findings which would indicate the need for mechanical ventilation would include a PO_2 below 50 mm Hg while the patient is on 60 percent oxygen, and a PCO_2 greater than 50 mm Hg with a Ph of 7.35, the latter strongly pointing to acute respiratory acidosis.

It is important to establish respiratory rate and pattern prior to establishing mechanical ventilation procedures, as these are indicative of cerebral dysfunction.

As the patient progresses and stabilizes, close observation of respiratory function must be maintained, especially in the comatose or minimally responsive patient. Pneumonia is often a cause of death after head injury in the comatose patient.[6,7] Some causes of pneumonia in the head injured patient include aspiration of feeding or oral secretions and infection. Bacterial pneumonia occurs frequently in patients with tracheostomies, since their upper airway is not able to filter out disease-causing organisms. Early intervention by the therapist emphasizing positioning, chest physical therapy, and oral motor stimulation to facilitate saliva management can limit the incidence of pneumonia.

Thermal Control

Hypothermia. An important part of the early assessment of the head injured patient is the assessment of his ability to maintain normal body temperature. This is often neglected in the initial assessment, unless the patient was known to have experienced a period of prolonged exposure. While hypothermia is usually caused by exposure to drugs (usually a sedative) or alcohol ingestion, it can also be indicative of Wernicke's Syndrome.[8]

Hyperthermia. Severe thermal regulation difficulties, such as those seen in dysfunction of the hypothalamus, result in extreme periods of hyperpyrexia. Jamieson[6] describes a clinical picture of hyperthermia which includes fever (to 42° C), piloerections, peripheral vasoconstriction, and circulatory collapse. Extreme prolonged temperature elevations can cause marked microscopic anoxic neuronal changes.[9]

These so called "central fevers" must be differentiated from fevers caused by other factors. Some causes of elevated temperature in the head injured patient include infection, deep vein thrombosis, and the presence of fat emboli. If cultures and other appropriate diagnostic studies are negative, then a diagnosis of central fever or hypothalamic dysfunction should be considered. In addition, it should be noted that recent studies are now showing that increased muscle spasticity will cause an increase in temperature.

Treatment of central fever includes standard treatment for pyria, such as antipyretics (aspirin [ASA] and acetaminophen) and cooling of the skin surface by hypothermia blanket. It is imperative to keep the body temperature at 38° C or less in order to prevent additional damage to brain tissue.

**Table 3-1. Symptomatology in Relation to
Probable Site of Dysfunction.**

Symptom	Site of Dysfunction
Jacksonian (focal, localized twitching)	Frontal lobe
Localized numbness	Parietal lobe
Lip smacking	Anterior temporal lobe
Olfactory hallucination	Posterior temporal lobe
Visual hallucination	Temporal or occipital lobes
Psychomotor	Temporal lobe

Seizures

Post-traumatic Seizures. Seizure activity can occur at any time after the initial trauma. While statistics vary as to the incidence of post-traumatic seizures,[10-12] patients who have open head injuries, intracranial hematomas, or who develop intracranial infection are most susceptible.[13] Post-traumatic seizures are generally classified as early or late onset. Early onset seizures are most common in children under five years of age, while in adults, seizures seldom occur without a depressed skull fracture, intracranial hematoma, or state of unconsciousness lasting more than several hours.

There are many types of seizure activity which can be exhibited by a patient, and any one patient may exhibit more than one type of seizure activity. Since symptomatology is often indicative of the area of dysfunction, it is important that an accurate description of both the manifestation and length of seizure is well documented. A table of frequently seen seizure activity and probable site of dysfunction is shown in Table 3-1.

In his study of post-traumatic seizures, Jeannett[12] notes that late onset seizures (more than one week post injury) will occur in approximately five percent of all patients who sustain blunt head injuries, with a significant increase in patients with skull fracture (early onset seizures, intracranial hematoma, or prolonged post-traumatic amnesia).

The use of prophylactic anticonvulsant medication remains a controversial subject among physicians. The two medications most frequently used, phenobarbital and phenytoin sodium (Dilantin®), often have sedating effects, which can mask symptoms of such complications as increased intracranial pressure. They can also cause difficulty in determining a patient's true level of awareness. A broad scale survey of American neurosurgeons showed only 60 percent used anticonvulsants prophylactically in the treatment of head injury.

When doing either an initial or follow-up assessment, it is important to note whether the patient is on anticonvulsant therapy. Should a change in the patient's level of awareness occur (increased lethargy, for example), blood levels and possible dosage change should be reviewed by the physician.

It should be noted that carbamazepine (Tegretol®) and valproic acid are now being used by some physicians and institutions for the treatment of post-traumatic seizure activity. Both drugs appear to have a much lower sedative effect at therapeutic levels.

EEG changes in patients exhibiting early post-onset seizure activity include widespread slow waves and suppression of normal frequencies, along with bursts of high voltage slow waves.[15] Unfortunately, the EEG cannot be used as a diagnostic tool in predicting which patients are at risk for developing late onset, post-traumatic seizures. EEG as an assessment tool will be further discussed in Chapter 4.

It may be of note to the therapist that in their initial study on the prognostic evaluation of the persistence of post-traumatic seizures, Weiss and Caveness[16] found that a patient who may have had only one seizure in the first week was not likely to have further seizures. To date, there is no indication that any treatment or therapy in the acute phase can reduce the incidence of seizures, as they are directly related to the amount of damage sustained at the time of injury.[17]

Increased Intracranial Pressure

Intracranial pressure is often significantly elevated in patients with head injury. Looking at the physiology of the brain and anatomy of the skull makes this easy to understand. Any change in either the brain itself, cerebral spinal fluid, or in the blood supply will cause a change in the other two. Increased intracranial pressure results from an addition to the volume in excess of the capacity.

Normal intracranial pressure (ICP) measures from 4 to 15 mm Hg. An intracranial pressure of greater than 20 mm Hg is considered abnormal and should be closely monitored. Intracranial pressure of 40 mm Hg causes neurologic dysfunction and impairment of the brain's electrical activity, as increased pressure limits the cerebral blood flow.[18]

Increased intracranial pressure tends to show a definite hierarchy of symptomatology. Most patients who are experiencing an increase in intracranial pressure complain of severe headache (providing the patient is cognitively able). This is usually followed by vomiting, though this is not necessarily projectile. Vomiting tends to occur more often after the patient awakes in the morning. Since the PCO_2 tends to be slightly increased in the morning, the cerebral artery blood flow is also increased.

As the intracranial pressure increases, there is a noticeable change in the

Table 3-2. Correlation of Physiologic Function, Level of
Consciousness, and Probable Site of Increased Intracranial Pressure.

Level of Consciousness	Respirations	Pupils	Probable Affected Area
Confused	Normal	Normal	Cerebrum
Stuperous	Periods of apnea (up to 60 sec.) followed by respirations of increasing depth & frequency (Cheyne-Stokes)	Small but reactive to light	Thalmus/ hypothalmus
Minimal to responsive	Cheyne-Stokes Prolonged hyperpnea	Midsized Nonreactive	Midbrain
Responsive	Irregular	Fixed or dilated	Medulla
Nonresponsive	Marked sustained inspiratory effort (apneusis)	Pinpoint Nonreactive	

patient's level of consciousness (Table 3-2). This can be either very gradual, such as a slight increase in lethargy, or very rapid. In the latter, a patient can go from alert to comatose in a matter of seconds, depending on how fast the pressure is rising and how severely the brain stem is being herniated. Cushing's Triad, in which blood pressure rises, and pulses and respirations significantly drop, will often be seen.

If the physician feels that the increased intracranial pressure is being caused by a hematoma, hygroma, or intracerebral hemorrhage, burr holes may be drilled in order to aspirate the fluid through a wide-bored brain cannula. Burr holes also allow for placement of ICP monitors, so that constant observation of changes in the intracranial pressure can be made.

If clinical symptoms suggest accumulation of fluid (hydrocephalus), a shunt may be performed. Shunts are often performed on patients with changes in level of consciousness when a CT scan indicates increasing enlargement of the ventricles.

If monitoring indicates changes in intracranial pressure, and the diagnosis of intracranial hematoma has been ruled out,[19] other treatment methods can be considered:

Dehydration: Many hospitals are now initiating the use of Lasix® as the primary dehydrating agent unless there is clinical indication of low serum osmology.[20] Mannitol is often given as a dehydrating agent. Close monitoring of serum osmology is necessary, as it can cause severe metabolic disorders.

Fluid restriction: Decrease fluids to two thirds to one half of the maintenance levels.

Hyperventilation: This will decrease the patient's PCO_2 level, thereby decreasing cerebral artery blood flow.

Positioning: Traditionally, the patient is positioned with the head of the bed at 30 to 40 degrees to allow for maximally effective blood flow. However, in recent literature, Raper, et al,[21] reported that 47 percent of patients had no change in intracranial pressure, or did not demonstrate a decrease in intracranial pressure when positioned flat in bed.

Cardiovascular Changes. Cardiovascular changes are often seen in the patient with increased intracranial pressure. As intracranial pressure rises, increased pressure causes compression to the medulla. The result is low blood pressure and rapid pulse. Other abnormalities of the cardiovascular system seen in the head injured patient with increased intracranial pressure are sinus arrhythmias and marked increase of pulmonary artery pressure due to increased pulmonary vascular arrhythmia.

Trauma to the vascular system itself at the time of the injury can result in thrombosis, occlusion, or aneurysm.

Thrombosis. Thrombosis due to trauma is often seen in the neck and base of the skull.[22] Symptoms often include hemiparesis or hemiplegia, with a noted unilateral sensory disturbance.[23]

Aneurysm. Aneurysms are frequently found in the patient with severe craniocerebral injury, including intracerebral hematoma and skull fracture. The aneurysm is most often located in the area of the wound. An aneurysm may also result from incomplete disruption of the arterial wall.

Occlusion. The areas most prone to occlusion appear to be the vertebral and basilar arteries. With their proximity to the skull and cervical spine, they are frequently compressed in hyper-extension injuries. Depending on the severity of the occlusion, symptomatology may be either rapid and abrupt onset of coma, or transient ischemic-like symptoms associated with decreased cerebral vascular perfusion.

Hypertension. Hypertension after head injury is a well known phenomenon and the incidence of this is estimated at 11 percent.[24] Unlike the patient with increased intracranial pressure who exhibits Cushing's Triad (refer to section on intracranial pressure), typically the head injured patient exhibits an elevation of systolic pressure, increased cardiac output, tachycardia, and abnormal or decreased peripheral vascular resistance.[24] Increased intracranial pressure has also been shown to cause prolonged increases in systemic pressure.

As in other vital body mechanisms, damage to the hypothalamus can also cause severe hypertension. A region in the posterior hypothalamus increases blood pressure and heart rate when stimulated. (Conversely, a region in the anterior hypothalamus lowers blood pressure when stimulated.[25]) Other possible causes of hypertension include renal failure and endocrine disorders.

Nutrition

Nutrition plays an important part in the patient's overall physiological recovery from severe head injury. While only a few clinical studies on nutrition have been done,[26-28] all indicate neurological injury increases metabolic expenditure. Kaln[29] notes that severe injury increases energy expenditure by 10 to 30 percent above resting levels, and sepsis may increase this by as much as 60 percent. Numerous factors affect increased metabolism, including hyperpnea, fever, spontaneous motor activity, and posturing.[30]

Conversely, it is important to note that barbituate and neuromuscular blocking agents may reduce the patient's metabolic rate by as much as 30 percent.[29] This should be of particular interest to the therapist working with the patient who is being treated with dantrolene sodium and baclofen, as he may not need as high a caloric intake as other patients and weight gain can prove to be a detriment to therapy.

In the patient not being treated with the above noted medications, caloric intake should be closely monitored to insure that an adequate caloric intake is maintained, as well as assuring the least nitrogen loss possible. The appropriate nutritional management of the head injury patient will result in the prevention of such complications as excessive tissue wasting, muscular weakness, organ dysfunction, and impaired or lost defenses,[31] all of which can severely impede any physical gains of which the patient may be capable.

Orthopedic Complications

Musculoskeletal Injury

Another complication of head injury that can significantly affect the ultimate functional outcome for the patient is musculoskeletal injury.[32-34] Since the majority of head injuries occur as a result of a motor vehicle accident or other traumatic event, many patients concomitantly sustain multiple injuries, including fractures, dislocations, and peripheral nerve damage.[33,35] Skeletal trauma associated with head injury has been reported to occur in 33 percent to 67 percent of victims, with most of these patients sustaining fractures or dislocations at more than one site.[36-41] These injuries may not be immediately diagnosed, because the patient may be unable to provide a history or indicate pain, and the immediate lifesaving techniques may preclude a complete physical and radiographic examination.[2,34,35]

Garland and associates[34,42] reported an 11 percent incidence of undetected musculoskeletal injuries. Therapists, nurses, or families who are in frequent contact with the patient may be the first to notice these injuries. Nerve damage may not be evident until there are clinical signs of muscle wasting or when the patient begins to awaken.[34] Early orthopedic intervention is critical to allow the patient to achieve his maximal functional recovery.[34] Garland and Bailey[42] found that neglected orthopedic care resulted in the most severe, permanent disability in patients who made good neurological recoveries. Therefore, injuries with a high incidence in this population should be sought out for optimal management.

Lower extremity fractures are more common, more easily missed, and more often associated with multiple fractures than upper extremity fractures.[34,43] Glenn and associates reported much higher mortality rates associated with combined head injury and femur fracture (20.6 percent) than with either head injury (12.0 percent) or- femur fracture (4.1 percent) alone.[38] Garland and Rhoades[43] reported incidences as high as 30 percent of all head injured patients sustaining upper extremity fractures, and 35 percent sustaining lower extremity fractures at more than one site. Most nerve injuries are associated with a fracture, but can also be the result of direct trauma.[42] The most common nerve damage associated with a lower extremity fracture occurs in the peroneal nerve.[35,42] The most common nerve damage associated with an upper extremity fracture occurs in either the ulnar or median nerve.[35,42] Any flail extremity should alert the therapist to the possibility of a peripheral nerve injury, and a flail upper extremity could be the result of a brachial plexus injury.[34,35,42]

Although the union rate for fractures sustained by head injured patients is the same as the normal population,[37,40,47] the management in this population may need to vary from traditional orthopedic approaches, giving careful consideration to neuromedical stability, motor manifestations, cognitive level, and ultimate outcome.[34,39,46] Orthopedic injuries in this population should be managed under the assumption that a full neurological recovery will be made.[33,39,43] Open reduction and internal fixation (ORIF) is frequently preferred over closed reduction and immobilization with slings, splints, casts, or traction when the patient is demonstrating restlessness, agitation, spasticity, or abnormal posturing (Table 3-3).[33-35,37,39,44,46]

With the restless or agitated patient, the presence of devices may increase agitation and the patient may remove or pull out external devices. Casts and appliances can be hazardous to the patient and staff when a patient is thrashing. Traction equipment will not allow adequate positioning of the spastic patient in reflex-inhibiting postures, and casts may not provide secure enough fixation against the pull of spastic muscles to prevent angulation or shortening of the fracture. Lower extremity fractures are reduced trying to maintain the length of

Table 3-3. Fixation Factors.

Internal Fixation	External Fixation
Unable to monitor neurologic status	Able to monitor neurologic status
Risks of anesthesia	No anesthesia
Early mobilization of affected extremity	Immobilization of affected extremity, depending on device
Rigid fixation cannot be removed by patient	Variable fixation—may be removable by patient
Early mobility of patient	May impede mobility of patient
Increased possibility of infection at site	Decreased possibility of infection at site
Will not cause injury to unaffected body parts	May cause injury to unaffected body parts
Increased ability to position patient	Limits ability to position patient
Anatomical alignment	Higher incidence of angulation
Maintains length	Higher incidence of shortening
Decreased chance of skin breakdown on affected extremity	Increase chance of skin breakdown on affected extremity (depending on fixation)

the extremity. In the head injured survivor, a 1 inch leg length discrepancy (which is acceptable and nonproblematic to the normal adult) may prevent functional ambulation when combined with the collective effects of sensory, motor, and balance deficits.

ORIF can provide the best means of maintaining length and at the same time allow for early mobilization. Early mobilization is essential to limit spastic contractures, limit the deconditioning effects of prolonged bedrest, and allow positioning for postural drainage and prevention of skin breakdown. ORIF is often recommended for patients with spasticity, but when casting is the treatment of choice, casts must be applied in neutral positions to prevent enhancement of spasticity and subsequent contractures.[34,35,38,41]

When a patient undergoes ORIF under general anesthesia, it is impossible to monitor neurological status, and any further decrease in status cannot be differentiated as a result of the head injury or anaesthesia and surgery.[33,34,39,46] Therefore, orthopedic surgery should be delayed until several hours to 24 hours of no change in the patient's neurological status.[2,33,39] The risks of anesthesia are minimized by seven to 10 days after the head injury, and this is the safest period for ORIF. A closed femoral fracture can wait this period; however, compound fractures, fractures with vascular injury, and primary suturing of tendons and nerves must be attended to as soon as possible.[2,33,39]

Better outcomes have been reported with ORIF of fractures of the femur, forearm, elbow, and shoulder in this population than with conventional methods[35,37-39,44-47] It is essential for the neurosurgeon and orthopedic surgeon to weight all the pros and cons neurologically, medically, and orthopedically to provide the best method of managing these complications.[2,33,39,46] Optimally, rehabilitation should begin in the acute surgical ward.[2]

Heterotopic Ossification

Heterotopic ossification (HO) is the growth of bone around joints for no apparent reason.[2,7,34-36] The first recorded development of heterotopic bone due to head injury was noted in 1968 by Roberts.[2] The etiology and pathophysiology is unclear[7,49-52] The disease is progressive and self-limiting,[49,52] and the process occurs in three steps: mineralization, calcification, and ossification.[53] Severe HO can result in the complete ankylosis of the affected joint.[51,53-55] The incidence of HO has been reported to be noted in 11 percent to 77 percent of patients with severe head injuries, and can involve multiple sites.[34,50,52,54,56] The ankylosis rate has been reported to be 16 percent and most commonly occurs in the elbow and hip.[34,54]

There are two types of HO found in the head injured population: traumatic and neurogenic (or ideopathic).[50] Traumatic HO occurs around a joint that has been traumatized by fracture or dislocation without any relationship to spasticity.[47,50] There is a possibility that ORIF is sufficient trauma to the joint to promote heterotopic bone formation.[53] Neurogenic HO occurs around joints that have not been injured.[50] The population at risk for neurogenic HO are those head injury victims who sustain diffuse axonal injury, coma of greater than two to four weeks duration, a Glasgow Coma Score of 3 to 8, spasticity, and immobility.[7,34,34,47,49,53-54,56,58] The onset generally ranges from one to nine months post head injury,[7,52,56] with the longest time documented after one year with a patient in a persistent vegetative state.[7,53] Clinical and radiographic evidence is most commonly documented at two months post onset of head injury (Figure 3-1).[34,52]

The clinical signs of HO are warmth, redness, pain, mild swelling, and decreased range of motion.[7,34,41,50,53,54] Thrombophlebitis must also be ruled out, as the signs and symptoms are similar.[41,53,59] Diagnostic studies include serum alkaline phosphatase, bone scan, and x-ray. HO should be suspected in this population with any of the clinical signs, or with an increase in the level of alkaline phosphatase in the bloodstream; however, increased blood levels are also noted with fractures, or with natural growth.[34,41] When clinical signs first appear, the bone scan and x-ray may still be negative.[34,41,51] A bone scan can show areas of increased uptake even with negative x-rays.[34,41,53]

The earliest diagnostic tool is the three phase bone scan described by Freed, et al,[59] in studying spinal cord injury patients. Increased vascularity can be seen in Phases I and II without a positive bone scan.[53,59] Technetium 99m (meth-

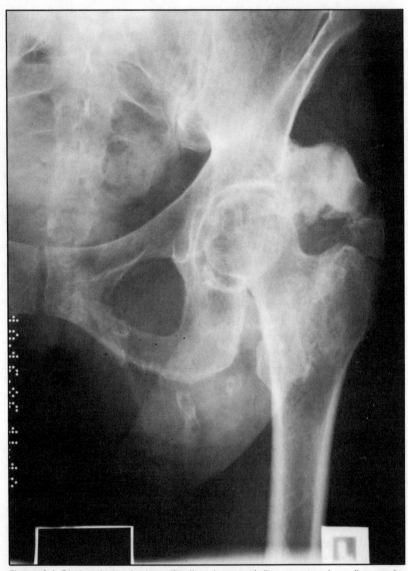

Figure 3-1. Obvious heterotopic ossification documentation on x-ray above the greater trochanter, significantly limiting abduction of the left hip. X-ray courtesy of Lake Erie Institute of Rehabilitation.

ylene diphosphonate) is injected and a dynamic blood flow study is done (Phase I); an immediate static scan is done to demonstrate a blood pool (Phase II); and a two hour bone scan is done to visualize accumulation of the radionuclide (Phase III-positive bone scan).[59] This study has been reported to be equally useful with head injured patients by Rogers.[53] See Table 3-4 for a summary of clinical and diagnostic signs of HO.

Just as the etiology and pathophysiology are unclear, so is the treatment. HO management has three phases: prevention, maintenance, and correction. HO can have a dramatically limiting effect on the head injured survivor, with complications of functional disability and a prolonged rehabilitation process. [34,36,53,54,56] Therefore, prevention is critical and time is the primary factor.[53]

Preventative treatment includes prophylactic disodium etidronate (Didronel®), passive range of motion, and spasticity limiting techniques. Didronel® must be started prior to the presence of any clinical or diagnostic signs. Although Spielman, et al,[56] indicated good results when the medication was initiated within two to seven days post onset of head injury, Rogers[53] reports that it is most effective when started within the first 24 hours post injury. The medication takes two weeks to achieve therapeutic levels at the recommended dosages of 20 mg/Kg/d for 12 weeks, followed by 10 mg/kg/d for 12 to 24 more weeks.[49,56,60,61] When administered after the onset of HO, Didronel® has been shown to slow the progression of the bone.[49]

Although there are numerous studies documenting the effectiveness of Didronel® in preventing HO and possibly retarding growth, there is no evidence of any effect on mature bone.[7,49,50,53,58] The only known side effect is diarrhea and this can be eliminated by administering the dose at half strength two times per day.[56,58] It is the responsibility of the care givers in the acute care stage to initiate preventative treatment.

Early physical therapy intervention of mobilization and inhibition of spasticity should be initiated as soon as possible. Garland, et al,[54] have correlated the exact location of the heterotopic bone to the site of spastic muscles (Table 3-5). The therapist should be alerted by the presence of spasticity and initiate appropriate positioning regimes, range of motion exercises, splinting, and casting. No increase in heterotopic bone has been documented as being caused by range of motion exercises.[50,51,53,55-67] Careful consideration should be made regarding early utilization of antispasticity medications[53] which are addressed later in this chapter. In patients at risk for developing traumatic HO (fracture or dislocation of elbow or hip, status post ORIF), continuous passive movement units may eliminate the effect of immobilization.[7,53] Garland and O'Hollaren[47] documented an 89 percent incidence of HO of the elbow with combined head injury and elbow fracture or dislocation.

Maintenance treatment is undertaken once HO is documented to limit any further loss of range of motion or function. Maintenance treatment may include antispasticity medications, passive range of motion (including CPM once

Table 3-4. Heterotopic Ossification in Head Injury.

Risk Factors	Clinical Signs	Diagnostic Studies	Common Sites	Ankylosis	Resection Outcome
1. Musculoskeletal trauma	1. Warmth	1. Serum alkaline phosphatase	1. Hip	1. High percentage	1. High percentage regrowth
2. Diffuse axonal injury	2. Redness	2. Bone scan	2. Elbow	2. High percentage	2. Low regrowth
3. Coma of greater than two to four weeks.	3. Decreased range of motion	3. X-ray	3. Shoulder	3. Small percentage	
4. Spasticity	4. Pain		4. Knee		
5. Immobility	5. Swelling				
6. ORIF					

Table 3-5. Formation of Heterotopic Bone Compiled
from Data Reported by Garland, et al.

Joint	Posturing	Location of Bone
Shoulder	Adducted and internally rotated	Inferomedially
Elbow	Flexion	Anteriorally
	Extension	Posteriorally
Hip	Adduction	Inferomedially
	Flexed and externally rotated	Anteriorally
Knee	No pattern	No pattern

location is documented), positioning, splinting, casting, and manipulation under anesthesia. Forced manipulation under anesthesia resulted in an increase in functional range of motion without any increase in heterotopic bone in a study conducted by Garland, et al,[35,50] Better results were obtained in cases of neurogenic HO than in traumatic HO.[50]

Corrective treatment is surgical resection and reinstitution of Didronel® therapy. It is recommended for patients who are making (or have made) good neurological recovery.[34,48] The complications of resection are sepsis, hemorrhage, and regrowth/reankylosis.[51] Resection should not be performed until the heterotopic bone is mature.[7,34,49,51,57,58]

Maturity is normally noted between 12 to 18 months post onset,[7,34,51] but occurs more rapidly in traumatic HO, and may be as early as six months post onset.[34] Maturity is determined by a true bone cortex radiographically, a serial decrease in activity on bone scan, and a lowering or normal alkaline phosphatase level.[17,53] Waiting for maturity decreases the risks and complications of resection. Garland and Keenan[34] reported good to excellent outcomes after resection of bone around the elbow, and poor to fair outcomes with bone around the hip.

Outcomes were better with traumatic HO than neurogenic HO, but the pattern was the same.[34] Didronel® at doses of 20 mg/kg/d for 16 to 20 weeks has been shown to be effective in preventing regrowth.[63] Patients with residual spasticity have a higher rate of recurrence.

Osteoporosis

Another secondary orthopedic complication that does not occur at the time of the initial injury is osteoporosis.[33,62] There are two types of osteoporosis that can occur in the head injured population: disuse and post-traumatic. Both types are the result of bone reabsorption exceeding bone deposition. Bone deposition is proportional to the stimulation of muscle pull and weight bearing.[62] Post-traumatic osteoporosis occurs in bones that are deprived of stress on the bones secondary to trauma.[62]

Disuse osteoporosis results from restricted activity and prolonged bedrest, is more generalized than post-traumatic osteoporosis, and is usually most marked in the lower extremities and spine.[62] Early physical therapy intervention and getting the patient out of bed as soon as possible can prevent or limit the process, as the stress on the bones can maintain the integrity of the skeletal system.[62] Weight bearing through all four extremities should also be initiated as soon as possible.

Intensive therapy with a gradual increase in the stresses applied can also reverse the process.[33,62] Whenever initiating therapy programs with patients who have been immobilized for extended periods of time, osteoporosis must be suspected, and care must be executed to limit the incidence of pathological fractures.[33]

Cognitive Deficits

The cognitive deficits which result from a severe closed head injury are, many times, even more devastating to the patient than physical deficits. While the patient may have a functional physical recovery, his cognitive deficits may preclude him from being able to function outside of a highly structured setting.

Many times the therapist unfamiliar with head injury will question his or her ability and expertise in dealing with the patient's cognitive problems and note that they are more comfortable dealing with the patient's physical and functional disabilities. We reply to them, what if you had to teach a patient who had been head injured to walk with two canes? You must explain to him how to sequence the movement of their canes and arm swing with proper hip swing and foot placement. If he has a receptive disorder, your concise instructions may make no sense to him; if he has a severe memory dysfunction, he may only recall your instructions for 10 to 15 seconds without constant cueing. As you can see, when there is damage to the brain, how the patient responds to stimuli and reacts to his environment is vastly altered. In this section, we will review some of the major areas of cognitive dysfunction seen in the head injured patient.

Levels of Consciousness

There are two major components of consciousness: arousal and awareness. Arousal is necessary for an individual to interact with his environment. It is the basic function which reflects activation of the reticular activating system (RAS) by somatosensory stimuli or innate motivational systems such as hunger.[63] Deficits in arousal can range from total unresponsiveness to loss of affectual responses. These are indicated by either spontaneous or responsive (to stimulation) eye opening. In this state, the patient is awake and responsive to environmental stimuli. Arousal may occur with only brainstem function. Awareness is distinguished from arousal in that awareness implies functional cerebral hemispheres and is manifested by cognition of self or the environment.[63]

Language Disorders

Brain injury can result in physical, psychological, behavioral, and cognitive handicaps. Cognitive deficits have been recognized as salient and sometimes permanent sequelae to the acute phase of a head injury.[63,64] The patient with a head injury can suffer from impairments in the cognitive processes of attention, concentration, memory, problem solving, analysis and synthesis of information, categorization, association, integration, abstract reasoning, and speed of processing. Because these cognitive abilities are involved in language formulation and processing, post closed head injury language dysfunction is influenced and in some cases created by cognitive dysfunction.[64]

Head injury can cause many language disturbances. Much literature indicates that head injured patients experience an initial period of a complete dissolution of language abilities, then gradually and spontaneously recapitulate the ontogeny of language and eventually attain "normal speech."[66-68] Victims of head injury manifest decreased receptive and expressive abilities similar to an aphasic patient, but the language disturbances associated with head injury are different from traditional aphasic syndromes.

Typically, head injured patients are disoriented to person, place, and time; confused; and concrete or inflexible in their thinking. In addition, these individuals demonstrate decreased judgment, reasoning, initiation, and inhibition. They are frequently impulsive and unaware of safety needs. These same behaviors are evident in receptive, integrative, and expressive language. With closed head injury, cognitive dysfunction appears, according to Hagen[65] in the patient's receptive and expressive language in the form of combinations of the following symptoms:

1. Decreased auditory comprehension;
2. Decreased visual and reading comprehension;
3. Expressive language that does not make sense;
4. Language expressions that are gramatically correct but not relevant to the question, statement, or discussion;
5. Lack of ability to inhibit verbal expressions;
6. Inappropriate ordering of words in sentences or inappropriate grammar;
7. Inability to recall specific words.

Although a head injured patient may have a specific language disorder such as word finding problems, the majority of the patient's language difficulties are due to the disruption of cognitive processes. Therefore, rehabilitation is a team effort directed toward cognitive reorganization. As a change in cognitive processing occurs, language disorganization decreases.

Memory

Memory is one of the cognitive processes, and a frequent complication following closed head injury is a disturbance in memory functioning. Memory is a very broad concept that encompasses a variety of different aspects. It is a complex, three-stage process consisting of an encoding stage (construction of internal representation), a storage stage (holding information over time), and a retrieval stage (a transfer of information from long-term storage to consciousness).[69] Therapists have found it helpful to identify different types of memory to assist in rehabilitation efforts. Immediate memory and delayed memory involve retention for a period of one to 60 minutes; recent memory concerns itself with events of preceding days or weeks; remote memory processes are those which may be disturbed following closed head injury.[67,68]

The head injured individual may demonstrate a variety of memory disorders. It is helpful for the therapist to remember the diversity of memory dysfunction when placing demands on a patient to perform specific tasks which might appear to be simple, routine activities. Although each patient is different due to the nature of the injury, memory dysfunction may be manifested in middle and late stages of recovery. The retrieval or recall of information is dependent on initiating, sustaining, and switching attention; recognition of relevant and irrelevant information; and rehearsal, organization, storage of information, and recall in an organized manner.[63] A memory problem may affect an individual's ability to follow simple commands or directions, recall family or friends' names, or remember the sequence for dressing or when to eat a meal. As one deals with the head injured patient, it is not uncommon to repeat, restate, or reiterate directions or requests. As the recovery process occurs, the number of reminders or repetitions the caregivers provide gradually decrease.

Ability for New Learning

Learning attempts to take advantage of that which is already known in order to graft on new material.[70] Patients with closed head injury have difficulty with cognitive processes of integration, analysis, and synthesis, which are components of learning. Due to the disruption of these processes, brain injured individuals tend to have much difficulty acquiring new information. With the disruption of new learning, the framework for therapy consists of providing structure in the environment; providing structured therapeutic tasks; and assisting the patient in the use of compensatory strategies when possible.

Behavioral/Psychosocial Problems

Behavior

Post head injury behavioral sequelae can be the most difficult area for the therapist working with the head injured patient to deal with. It is probably the most difficult area to understand, diagnose, treat, and even predict. There are many factors that relate to and contribute to behavioral problems in the head injured patient.

The site of the lesion is primary. Damage to the frontal lobe is a significant factor in behavior problems or behavioral dysfunction. The frontal lobes appear to be the "regulators" of integrative behavior. A patient who sustains a frontal injury often behaves in a manner which makes no sense to the observer. Abilities such as being able to attend to a task, initiate activity, or participate in goal-directed behavior are significantly impaired.

Other areas of the brain, when traumatized, can cause significant behavioral problems. Damage to the temporal lobe structures may cause a patient to exhibit verbal or physical outbursts. Appetite disturbances, irritability, and mood swings have been seen in patients with damage to the hypothalamus.

It needs to be noted that a patient need not have a specific focal injury to exhibit behavioral changes. Problems such as depression, poor frustration tolerance, and sexual dysfunction are frequently seen in patients with diffuse, widespread damage.[71]

In addition to site of injury, other factors affecting neuropsychological functioning of the patient include premorbid level of functioning, severity of injury, age, and education.[72] The interaction of these factors is probably responsible for the vast behavioral differences seen in patients with closed head injury. A study done by Dikmen and associates[72] found that the severity of the injury (depth and duration of coma) is a greater factor in neurobehavioral deficits than post-traumatic amnesia.

Sexual Dysfunction

Unfortunately, little has been written to date on sexual dysfunction and disorders of the head injured patient. While sexual dysfunction in the head injured patient is most likely to be caused by damage to the temporal or frontal lobes, any disruption of the nervous system, i.e., head injury, can disrupt adequate and socially approved sexual behavior.[73]

Frequently seen disorders include inappropriate advances to staff members of the opposite sex, exposure, perseveration, and either decreased or increased sexual drive. Other physical and cognitive deficits such as confusion, short attention span, and poor memory only serve to compound the problems.

These disorders affect not only the patient, but the spouse or significant other as well. They are often confused by the patient's new behaviors, and the patient or significant other is often fearful of asking for help in coping.

While the therapist may not feel comfortable with providing counseling in this area, he or she needs to be aware of the problems of the sexually dysfunctional patient. The therapist can, however, help the patient cope with his body image and encourage self-control of inappropriate behavior through behavior management activities.

Social Problems

Socialization occurs as an interactive process of environmental conditions, cognitive development, and social/affective maturation.[74] In the head injured person, the ability for this interactive process is disrupted, usually by a combination of cognitive and physiological factors influencing this disruption, including age at time of injury, location of injury (see earlier discussion), severity of damage and length of coma, and premorbid personality.

When an individual suffers a head injury, the ability to functionally use social skills is impaired or lost, thus causing a disruption of the patient's ability to interact appropriately with his environment and with those within it. Frequently, the patient's own frustration with this inability only serves to increase the inappropriateness of his socialized behavior or skills. A carefully structured, consistent treatment plan is indicated for the patient who is exhibiting problems in the area of socialization.

The understanding of the behavioral sequelae of head injury is extremely important to the therapist in the planning of therapeutic activities and assessment of the patient's abilities and disabilities. The therapist's approach to the patient should be based on management of the behavioral problem(s).

In the patient who is confused or disoriented, the therapist will need to reorient the patient as needed, sometimes several times during a session. Patience and provision of information in a calm, nonthreatening manner will help prevent (or at least modify) the acting out or aggressive behavior often seen in the highly confused patient.

The patient who is easily overstimulated may need to be seen in a small, quiet area where distractions are at a minimum. Allow the patient to relax if he appears to become overstimulated. Remember to present only one stimulus item at a time when working with this patient. This type of patient may become agitated if overstimulated.

Neuromotor Dysfunction

Neuromotor dysfunction secondary to traumatic head injury generally has a more favorable prognosis for recovery than cognitive ability and is less limiting to the patient with regard to ultimate functional outcome and independence. Impairments are common in motor control, which can be viewed as the interaction of sensory and perceptive functions. Some of these are amenable to treatment, some of these will remain as residual deficits. This section deals with neuromotor impairments that are a direct result of head injury. Physical limitations that arise post head injury (i.e., contractures secondary to spasticity and immobilization) will be addressed in the sections on assessment and treatment.

Sensation

Sensation is comprised of all input coming from the environment. All sensory modalities may be altered by head trauma and may be manifested by a total loss of or alteration in sensation.

Sensation can be divided into three categories: gross sensation, cortical sensation, and the special senses. The gross sensations include touch, pressure, position, temperature, and pain. Cortical sensations encompass stereognosis, graphesthesia, simultaneous tactile sense, and two-point discrimination. The special senses are sight, smell, taste, and hearing. These special senses are most frequently impaired, and most disabling following head injury.

Interruption of sensation can occur at any level of the afferent pathways from the receptors to the brain, and given the nature of head injury, probably occurs at multiple levels.

The most severe level of sensory dysfunction, the inability to receive or process sensory information, prevents interaction with the environment. Some sensory deficits will subside with spontaneous recovery, and treatment is aimed at stimulating the sensory system to aid recovery. The only available treatment of residual sensory dysfunction is education of the patient to compensate for specific losses. Sensory dysfunction will affect the head injured patient's perceptual and motor abilities, thereby interfering with functional abilities. Controlled movement is dependent upon sensory feedback from the part being moved.

Perceptual Dysfunction

Perception is the system by which sensory information is organized. Perceptual dysfunction is a frequent complication in the head injured patient. Due to the often diffuse nature of injury, many perceptual pathways can be damaged, causing the patient to be unable to accurately perceive and integrate input from sensory modalities. Some of the functions affected include: somatosensory functions, visual awareness, and position in space.

Visual deficits are among the most common of the perceptual dysfunctions. These include impaired focusing and tracking in the low level patient, impaired ability to cross the visual midline, impaired depth perception, and diplopia. The patient with agnosia loses the organizational and perceptual synthesis of sensation. Most often, it is a disturbance in the recognition of objects in a specific sensory mode. The most commonly seen agnosias in the head injured patient are visual, visuospatial, tactile, and distortion of the spatial image of the body.

Body image distortions are also common in the patient with perceptual dysfunction. Here, the patient is either unaware of body parts or has a misconception of its position. Unilateral neglect in which the patient ignores one side of his body, even when there is no weakness or sensory loss, is often seen.

Any of these dysfunctions, singly or in combination, will affect the patient's motor abilities and functional skills.

Spasticity

Spasticity is a very common motor complication of head injury,[33,75-77] and is one of the most common lingering disorders that compromises functions. It is the result of the disruption of the balancing influences of descending inhibitory and facilitatory tracts[78-81] or deficient spinal inhibitory mechanism[80] causing excessive stimulation of alpha/motor neurons[80] most frequently due to the release of the gamma system from higher inhibitory control.[77-79,82,83] This disruption is in response to lesions anywhere along the pathways of the extrapyramidal system, the reticular activating system, the basal ganglia, the cerebellum, the cerebral cortex, internal capsule, brain stem, and spinal cord[33,84-87] and results in the hypersensitivity of muscle spindles.[79,86] Spasticity is mediated through the spindle afferents at the reflex level.[79,85,86] The reflex pathway that supports the spastic state is the lateral vestibular nucleus and lateral vestibular tract.[85] Pathways facilatory to antigravity muscles stay intact because they are not dependent on higher centers (lateral reticulospinal tract and lateral vestibulospinal tract), whereas the inhibitory system (corticobulbar, lenticulobulbar, cerebroreticular, and medial reticulospinal tracts) is dependent on higher centers.[85]

Spasticity is frequently described by the degree of resistance a muscle group gives in response to stretch,[82,83,85,87,88] and can be defined as a state of hypertonicity or striated skeletal muscles as manifested by increased resistance to passive stretch due to increased responses of static and phasic stretch reflexes.[79,80,77,83,87,88]

Bishop[79] describes a triad of motor signs associated with spasticity which are hyperactive phasic stretch reflexes, hyperactive tonic stretch reflexes, and clonus.

The clinical signs of hyperactive tonic stretch reflexes include the clasp-knife response (or lengthening reaction), progressive resistance to passive movement, and velocity dependent resistance to movement.[77,80,82,87,89] When the spastic muscles are subjected to passive stretch, the amount of resistance to that movement progressively increases throughout the movement.[77,80,87] The resistance may suddenly subside as the movement approaches the limit of range of motion (clasp-knife response or lengthening reaction).[77,80,87] The early and mid-period produces greater resistance, whereas the later and terminal period produces relaxation.[77,85] The degree of resistance is dependent upon and proportional to the velocity of movement. Slower movement elicits minimal resistance, and faster movement elicits maximal resistance.[77,80]

The clinical signs of hyperactive phasic stretch reflexes (hyperreflexia) are an increase in the response of the tendon reflex (i.e., responds with decreased stimulus), and a reflex response of neighboring muscles which were not stimulated.[77,79,80,82,87,90]

Clonus is repeated contractions of a muscle in response to quick stretch which frequently appears with spasticity, but is not an invariable component.[77,80]

Spasticity is highly variable in individual patients as is the response to various treatment approaches in similar patients.[80,91]

There are two types of spasticity: alpha and gamma. Although both types are a result of increased drive to the alpha motor neuron, gamma spasticity is a result of the gamma spindle loop affect on the alpha motor neuron resulting from loss of inhibition of the gamma system.[77,80] Alpha spasticity is a result of loss of supraspinal inhibition of alpha motor neurons.[77,79] Gamma spasticity can be defined as spasticity which decreases or is eliminated by interruption of the gamma spindle loop.[77,79] Alpha spasticity is spasticity that is unchanged with interruption of the gamma loop.[77,79] These two types are spasticity responding differently to various interventions, and these can be differentiated clinically by application of cold.[77,79] Gamma spasticity diminishes in response to cold; alpha spasticity remains the same or increases.[77,79]

In head trauma, there are widespread cerebral or brainstem lesions involving the descending inhibitory pathways and resulting in hyperactivity of both alpha and gamma motor neurons.[77] Therefore, many head injured patients present with a mixed form of spasticity.[77,83] Some muscles may present with gamma spasticity and others with alpha spasticity. Cerebral spasticity is generally more regular than spinal cord spasticity.[77,87] It is heavily influenced by postural changes and body positioning.[75,77,82,85-88] It is frequently enhanced by abnormal tonic reflex activity at the spinal and brainstem levels.[33,77,87,92] It is frequently more pronounced distally than proximally, and is usually seen in combination with other motor manifestations.[79]

Spasticity often partially or totally masks voluntary movement.[75,77,83,87] When movement is present, it is usually characterized by stereotyped, synergistic patterns associated with co-contraction of antagonist muscles resulting in a lack of isolated movement.[77,83] When isolated movements are present, they are frequently uncoordinated, slow, and stiff.[77] Attempts at maximal voluntary contractions in a spastic extremity can frequently result in a movement opposite of the movement intended.[77,87] A voluntary contraction of an unaffected extremity can result in a similar, "mirrored," movement of the affected extremity, known as an associated reaction or movement.[77,87,93] Spasticity in head trauma can be seen in the absence of attempted movement, in the presence of attempted movement, and as an inability to relax after performing a movement.[77,87]

The negative effects of spasticity include sensations of pain or tightness, sleeplessness, contractures, subluxations, dislocations, postural deformities, interference with hygiene and skin care, interference with functional movement, and reinforcement of abnormal movement.[75,78,85,88,92,94]

The positive effects of spasticity include maintenance of muscle bulk, retardation of the development of osteoporosis, facilitation of circulation, and possible assistance in stand/pivot transfers.[61,75,94]

Spasticity is also enhanced by environmental factors such as excessive sensory input, emotional stress, changes in external temperature, and internal factors such as pain, infection, and changes in internal temperature.[85,94]

Treatment must be aimed at breaking up a spastic cycle, i.e., spasticity causes pain and pain increases spasticity, tonic reflexes enhance spasticity and spasticity enhances tonic postures. Numerous interventions are available but empirical, with a lack of scientific documentation of results. Presently, spasticity is most frequently subjectively evaluated and rated as resistance to passive stretch and interference with functional activity. Therefore, the response to any given treatment procedure is documented in the same way.[90,95]

The management of spasticity can be divided into pharmacologic, therapeutic, and surgical interventions.[77,91] Centrally acting drugs preferentially depress small neurons in the lateral reticular formation which have facilitatory control over spinal motoneurons.[91] However, in the process of depressing the descending facilitatory pathways, these drugs also depress the ascending reticular system which is responsible for arousal or wakefulness.[91] Therefore, a major side effect of these medications is lethargy and sedation.[77,91,96]

The sedative effect may cause an increase in respiratory depression, hypotension, difficulty handling secretions, muscle weakness, and dysphagia.[77,96] Centrally acting medications also have an effect on the cognitive areas of attention, memory, and confusion.[96]

Careful consideration of side effects along with close monitoring of effectiveness are necessary when utilizing antispasticity medications in the head injured population, as these patients already present with significant cognitive and physical deficits and may not be able to tolerate an enhancement of these deficits.[96] On the other hand, spasticity can significantly interfere with the

Table 3-6. Medications Commonly Utilized in Control of Spasticity.

Medication	Mechanism and Site of Action	Side Effects	Indications	Precautions/ Complications	Dosage
Diazepam (Valium*)	1. Inhibits the contraction mechanism of skeletal muscles 2. Enhances inhibition mediated at the spinal cord by enhancing alphaaminobutyric acid presynaptic inhibition at the interneuron pool 3. Depresses the reticular activating system	1. Sedation/ drowsiness 2. Dizziness 3. Ataxia 4. Muscle weakness 5. Habituation 6. Potential respiratory depression 7. Potential dysphagia 8. Decreased attention 9. Decreased memory	1. Most effective with spasticity due to brainstem or spinal cord lesions 2. Beneficial when sedation is desirable (i.e., agitation)	1. May complicate management of seizures 2. Abrupt withdrawal may severely intensify spasticity	25 mg. q.d. or b.i.d. to start Gradually and cautiously increased depending on primary and secondary effects. Pediatric max. 5 mg. q.i.d.
Ketazolam	Same as diazepam (Valium*)	Same as diazepam but to lesser extent	1. Relaxation of spasticity equal to diazepam 2. Can be given in one dose 3. May be drug of choice if greatest spasticity is at night		50-60 mg. q.d.
Baclofen (Lioresal*)	Enhances inhibition mediated at the spinal cord and brainstem levels by enhancing alpha aminobutyric acid presynaptic inhibition at the interneuron pool	1. Sedation (less than diazepam) 2. Anorexia 3. Nausea 4. Vomiting 5. Dizziness 6. Constipation 7. Confusion 8. Decreased attention	1. More effective with alpha spasticity 2. More effective with spasms that impede voluntary effort 3. Useful with cerebral spasticity alone 4. Can be used in combination with dantrolene sodium (Dantrium*)	1. Rebound intensification of spasticity 2. Hallucinations on withdrawal 3. Possible hepatotoxicity	5 mg. t.i.d. w/ gradual increase every 3-4 days, up to 20 mg. q.i.d. (Some reports higher) Pediatric max. 20 mg. q.i.d.
Dantrolene Sodium (Dantrium*)	Facilitates release of calcium from the sarcoplasmic reticulum in striated muscles, blocking the excitation-contraction mechanism within the muscle fiber	1. Drowsiness (subsides with continued use) 2. Muscle weakness 3. Liver toxicity 4. Gastrointestinal complaints 5. Potential respiratory depression 6. Potential dysphagia	1. Most effective with alpha spasticity 2. Useful in combination with either diazepam or baclofen	1. Contraindicated in liver disease or dysfunction—routine hepatic studies necessary with all patients 2. Photic sensitivity 3. Long-term use may produce facial acne	25 mg. q.d. or b.i.d. gradually inc. to 400 mg./day Pediatric max. 25 mg. q.i.d.

patient's rehabilitation program. In the patient with limited attentional skills and severe spasticity, the patient may only attend to the physical discomfort of the spasticity, and be unable to interact with his environment and therapy.

A combination of dantrolene sodium, which acts best on alpha spasticity with the least effect on cognitive function, and either baclofen or diazepam, which acts best on gamma spasticity, may be the most appropriate centrally-acting pharmacologic approach to the management of spasticity by allowing the lowest possible dosages and affecting the mixed pattern of spasticity commonly seen with head injury (Table 3-6).

An effective method of managing spasticity is neurolysis, either peripheral nerve or intramuscular, utilizing injection of diluted phenol solution.[34,77,98-101] Nerve blocks can be performed by an open surgical method or a closed percutaneous method.[34,77,97,99,99] Open methods are used when the nerve to be injected contains both sensory and motor components.[34,98] The motor branches are identified with the aid of a nerve stimulator to spare the sensory component[36] and prevent sensory loss and dysethesias.[34,98] Nerve blocks result in complete cessation of muscle activity and may be indicated with severe spasticity[34,98] The benefits last from four to six months.[34,98,99] Therapeutic methods of facilitating voluntary movement, including application of casts, splints, and braces should also be utilized during this time to enhance the functional benefits.[34,77,98-101] Most of the patients to have shown prolonged benefits (greater than six months) from motor nerve block had selective motor control of their spastic muscles prior to treatment.[79] Common side effects are local pain, swelling, and edema, which usually subside within several days after the injection.[97]

Dyesthesias can commonly occur when mixed motor and sensory nerves are injected at the level of the peripheral nerve, plexus, or root.[97] These dyesthesias begin several days after injection and last for approximately a week.[97]

Intramuscular neurolysis involves locating the motor points of the spastic muscle group with a stimulator and percutaneously injecting the motor points with a phenol solution.[34,101] Motor point blocks do not give complete cessation of muscle activity and may be indicated with mild spasticity.[34] The side effects include transient muscle pain and formation of fibrotic nodules.[77]

Therapeutic intervention is aimed at simultaneously inhibiting the spastic antagonist and facilitating the agonist, and progresses to facilitation of a smooth reversal of antagonists. There are a number of inhibition and facilitation techniques available to the therapist that include hands-on techniques and modalities. Table 3-7 summarizes elements of treatment that lead to a reduction of spasticity or an increase in voluntary movement.[102] Many of these techniques are based on providing peripheral stimulation which travels along multiple loop pathways to increase or decrease excitability of spinal motoneurons to reduce spasticity or enhance voluntary movement.[103] Some inhibitory elements provide a generalized decrease in tone, while others result in a localized decrease in tone in the muscle or muscle group stimulated.

A generalized decrease in tone can be obtained through rhythmical rocking, slow stroking down the posterior primary rami, stimulation of the carotid sinus by lowering the patient's head, neutral warmth, visual simulation, and auditory stimulation.[102,104,105]

A localized decrease in tone can be obtained through facilitation of the antagonist, vibration of the antagonist, maintained stretch, pressure on long tendons, light touch with resistance, and quick ice with resistance.[102,104-111]

Table 3-7. Inhibition and Facilitation Techniques.

I. Generalized Response

Stimulus	Response
1. Slow stroking down posterior primary rami	1. Generalized relaxation
2. Vestibular stimulation:	2. a. Generalized facilitation of phasic responses
a. Angular or transient linear acceleration	b. Generalized facilitation of tonic responses
b. Maintained linear acceleration	3. a. Generalized relaxation
3. Rocking	b. Generalized facilitation and arousal
a. Slow, rhythmical	4. Relaxation
b. Rapid, irregular	5. Generalized relaxation
4. Neutral warmth	6. a. Facilitation/arousal
5. Carotid sinus reflex	b. Generalized relaxation
6. Visual	7. a. Facilitation/arousal
a. Bright, moving	b. Generalized relaxation
b. Dim	
7. Auditory	
a. Loud, irregular	
b. Soft, regular	

II. Localized Response

Stimulus	Response
1. Rhythmical rotation	1. Relaxation of part being moved
2. Neutral warmth	2. Relaxation of part being wrapped
3. Visual	3. Facilitation of desired response
4. Verbal commands	4. Facilitation of desired response
5. Vibration	5. Facilitation of agonist, inhibition of antagonist
6. Approximation/bone pounding	6. Facilitation of tonic response in muscles around stimulated joint
7. Brushing	7. Facilitation of tonic response in muscles stimulated
8. Maintained touch	8. Facilitation of tonic response in muscles touched
9. Light touch:	9. a. Facilitation of phasic response in muscle touched
a. With resistance	b. Inhibition of phasic response in muscle touched
b. Without resistance	10. Facilitation of phasic response in muscles surrounding stimulated joint
10. Traction	11. Facilitation of phasic response in stretched muscle
11. Quick stretch	12. Inhibition of stretched muscle
12. Maintained stretch	13. Inhibition of stimulated muscle
13. Pressure on tendons	14. a. Facilitation of phasic response in muscle stimulated
14. Quick ice:	b. Inhibition of phasic response in muscle stimulated
a. With resistance	15. a. Facilitation of tonic response in resisted muscles
b. Without resistance	b. Overflow/irradiation
15. Resistance	
a. Graded	
b. Maximal	

Table 3-8. Suggested Uses of Cold in Treatment of Spasticity.

Method	Temperature	Duration
Wet towels with crushed ice	10 °C 40 °F	10 minutes Two to three minutes; Replace every three hrs.
Immersion of limb	10 °C 50 °F 35 to 40 °F 60 to 65 °F 55 °F	10 minutes Five minutes Three to five minute dip; then out 15 to 20 minutes; repeat three to four times 10 to 20 minutes
Immersion of body	26.6 °C 50 °F 70 to 80 °F	20 minutes Four minutes 30 to 45 minutes
Ice packs	55 °F	10 to 15 minutes 20 minutes

Positioning has a significant effect on spasticity and prevention of contracture, and will be addressed in Chapter 5.

There are several modalities aside from therapeutic exercise techniques that can be utilized to control spasticity. These include cold, electrical stimulation, biofeedback, casting, splinting, and bracing.

Cold is thought to decrease the firing of muscle spindle afferents by raising the spindle threshold via direct cooling of the muscle[117] or through reflex cooling of the muscle via the sympathetic nervous system. Cold treatment can be provided by cold baths, cold packs, ice towels, ice/cold dips, or sprays (ethyl chloride, fluromethane).[102,105,112,113] Inconsistent responses to cold have been reported between affected and unaffected limits in hemiplegia patients, as well as inconsistencies from patient to patient.[86,91] Therefore, each patient must be individually evaluated for the desired response. Duration of effect may range from during treatment sessions up to 24 hours. Varying methods of application of cold are outlined in Table 3-8. Close monitoring is necessary during treatment to prevent a rebound effect of increased spasticity. A small area should be tested for hypersensitivity prior to treatment.

Electrical stimulation can be used to fatigue the spastic muscle or to facilitate the antagonist to the spastic muscle.[114] When utilizing electrical stimulation to spastic muscles, there should be a slow rise time and a prolonged on time to prevent quick stretch.[114] Short-term results are usually obtained lasting a few minutes to several hours.[77,114]

Electromyographic biofeedback can be used to retrain the patient to relax spastic muscles and move antagonistic muscles.[77,115,116] It is generally recommended to relax the spastic muscle first, prior to muscle re-education.[115] This can be accomplished by learning to relax the spastic muscle in a resting position and then progressing to keeping the relaxation while placing motoric demands on other body parts when using the affected extremity after stretch and adding images of emotionally stressful situations.[115]

Casting, splinting, and bracing are all alternatives with varying degrees of spasticity. Bracing is usually deferred until a prediction of functional outcome can be made, most frequently in the rehabilitation facility. Splinting may be appropriate with mild to moderate spasticity. A variety of splints can be utilized to decrease tone or prevent contracture from spasticity. Resting pan splints maintain wrist and fingers in a functional position. Abductor splints for the fingers and abductor wedges for the lower extremities may diminish extensor tone in a generalized manner. Hard hand cones may decrease finger flexor spasticity via GTOs by providing maintained pressure on long tendons.

Posterior foot splints are generally contraindicated in head injury patients secondary to skin breakdown, and frequent equinovarus posturing that cannot be well controlled with these splints. Footboards are also not recommended. Firm hi-top sneakers may prevent contracture development by maintaining neutral alignment and preventing stimulation to the plantarflexor muscles. Variable position knee immobilizers, air splints, and dynasplints are all useful adjuncts to the treatment of spasticity.

Casting is being utilized in most head injury rehabilitation facilities and in some acute care hospitals. Casting provides maintained stretch, neutral warmth and elimination of facilitatory stimuli to decrease spasticity as well as maintain position. Serial casting is recommended when a patient has already lost passive range of motion secondary to increased tone. Positional assisting is recommended in the presence of plasticity without loss of range of motion.

Casts are changed every three to 10 days, depending on the facility's protocol. A bivalved cast can be utilized to prevent deformity in the presence of spasticity without loss of passive range of motion. Specific casting procedures will be addressed in Chapter 5 on treatment techniques.

Hypotonia/Flaccidity

Hypotonia is usually a transient state characterized by decreased tendon reflexes and loss of movement following head injury or surgery to the brain.[117] Hypotonia may also be the result of cerebellar damage and is characterized by brisk tendon reflexes, a pendular response to tendon tap, decreased response to passive movement, and decreased postural stability.[117]

Facilitation techniques must be used with care, as most patients with hypotonia post head injury eventually develop spasticity.[117] Facilitation should be aimed at developing postural control and normal movement patterns.

A generalized increase in tone can be facilitated by irregular, accelerating rocking, bright lights, brisk verbal commands, noxious odors, and light touch.[102,111,113]

A localized increase in tone can be facilitated with quick stretch, traction, light touch, maintained touch, visual input, verbal commands, vibration, approximation, and brushing.[102,111,113]

Rigidity

Another common neuromotor complication of head injury is rigidity which is generally seen in the form of decerebrate or decorticate posturing.[76] Classic decorticate posturing consists of flexion posturing in the upper extremities, and extensor posturing in the lower extremities.[77] Classic decerebrate posturing consists of extensor posturing of both the upper and lower extremities.[77] Head injured patients may have mixed forms of these postures and may fluctuate from one posture to another.[77] Rigidity is a form of hypertonus in which these characteristic postures are accompanied by increased resistance to passive stretch that is constant throughout.[77] Patients who respond to painful stimuli with decorticate or decerebrate postures have an increased mortality and morbidity rate compared to those patients who localize or withdraw from pain.[118] Decerebrate and decorticate rigidity may be seen in combination with spasticity after head injury, and this usually resolves to spasticity or disappears.[76]

Reflexes

Head injured patients also present with abnormal postural reflexes[33] when the tonic neck and labyrinthine reflexes are released from cortical control.[117] The presence of tonic reflexes prevents normal righting and equilibrium reactions.[92] Tonic neck reflexes are mediated by proprioceptors in the proximal cervical area and tonic labyrinthine reflexes are mediated by the vestibular system.[106] Both types of tonic reflexes result in a change in muscle tone in response to head movement or posture.[104]

Treatment is aimed at inhibiting primitive brainstem reflexes while facilitating higher level righting and equilibrium reactions.[92]

Movement Disorders

There are a multitude of movement disorders associated with head injury. Along with spasticity and hemiparesis, the most common lingering disorders that compromise functions are ataxia, bradykinesia, and tremors.

Ataxia is characterized by discoordinate, dysynergic movement and faulty balance.[76] It is frequently associated with hypotonia.[117] Dysnergia is deficient control of speed or timing of different muscle groups contracting in proper sequence.[89] Dysmetria is deficient control of position, direction, or distance of movement.[89] Limb ataxia is characterized by a decreased ability to coordinate smooth movements.[33] Truncal ataxia is characterized by a wide-based, unsteady gait with staggering upon turning.[33] Ataxia is the result of damage to the cerebellum or its connecting pathways.

Tremors are predictable, timed involuntary movements that occur at rest, with movement, or both, and that are often seen with upper motor neuron lesions.[76,119] These involuntary contractions of reciprocally innervated muscles produce rhythmic oscillations which may be alternating or synchronous and frequently take the form of rhythmic flexion and extension, supination, and pronation, or abduction and adduction.[119] Tremors may become prominent during the maintenance of sustained antigravity posture or during directed performance of a limb.[119]

The tremor may occur on the initiation of a movement with the amplitude of the tremor increasing as the limb approaches a target.[33,119] Tremors are regular and therefore can be distinguished from cerebellar ataxia that results in an irregular, nonpatterned incoordination of movement. Tremors can result from damage to the cerebellum or basal ganglia[33,84] and are combined with ataxia or spasticity after head injury.[33]

Apraxia

Another common motor disorder is the lack of ability to plan and execute a motor task, or apraxia.[96] Apraxia is characterized by the inability to perform a skilled movement on request even though the movement can be produced spontaneously.[87] Apraxia is an inability to organize motor output secondary to interpretation of perceptual information in the areas of body scheme, tactile sensory processing, and proprioception.[96]

In motor apraxia, there is a loss of kinesthetic memory patterns which results in a defect in execution and an inability to carry out a complicated sequence.[84] Simple tasks may be performed automatically.[84]

Ideomotor apraxia is the inability to imitate gestures or perform motor tasks on command.[84] The patient presents with motor planning problems with a loss of skilled sequence of movement and perseveration of movement.[84] The patient may be able to carry out overlearned tasks automatically.[84]

Ideational apraxia is the inability to perform an aotivity automatically or on command, although simple, isolated activities or parts of activities may be performed.[84] The patient cannot understand the concept of the activity, has difficulty with abstract commands, is unable to relate object names and visual images to a related motor activity, and is unable to describe the purpose of an object.[84]

Constructional apraxia is an inability to produce designs in two or three dimensions either on command or spontaneously, which limits the patient's ability to perform purposeful acts using objects in the environment.[120]

Verbal apraxia is the inability to form and organize intelligible words in the presence of intact musculature.[120]

Dressing apraxia is the inability to dress oneself secondary to a disorder in body scheme or spatial relations.[120]

Dyskinesias

Other than bradykinesia and athetosis, the dyskinesias are rarely seen in head injured patients, and when seen, may be the consequence of tranquilizing medications.[76]

Bradykinesia is slowed movement, either in the initiation or performance of a movement.[117] In head injury, bradykinesia is usually seen as a component of other neuromotor disorders.[76]

Dystonia presents as a relatively fixed and abnormal posture resulting from abnormal contraction of antagonistic muscles.[87,117] It is a severe form of hypertonus.[117,119] Dystonic movements are generally sustained twisting movements of varying speed which sustain postures at the height of the involuntary movement and overflow into remote muscles not usually used for the voluntary movement.[87,119] Dystonia can occur in association with athetosis.[119] In head injury, dystonia usually begins at rest, is nonprogressive, and frequently stabilizes as a unilateral dystonia.[119]

Athetosis is characterized by random, purposeless movements combined with postural instability.[117] Athetoid movements are continuous, slow, writhing movements that are involuntary and distal in distribution.[87,117,119]

Choreiform movements are irregular, continuous, unpredictable, non-repetitive, involuntary movements that are proximal in distribution and give the appearance of restlessness or fidgetiness.[87,119]

Ballismus is a form of chorea characterized by wild, involuntary flailings of the extremities.[87,119]

References

1. Chusia JG, McDonald J: Coma. In Correlative Neuroanatomy and Functional Neurology. Ed 17. Large Med Pales, Los Altos, Calif, 1979.
2. Jeannett B, Teasdale G: Management of Head injury. FA Davis Publishers, Philadelphia, 1981.
3. Jeannett B, Teasdale, G: Assessment of coma and impaired consciousness. Lancet 1974;2:81.
4. Brink JD, Imbus C, Woo-Sam J: Physical recovery after severe closed head trauma in children and adolescents. J Pediatr 1980;97:721.

5. Plum F, Posner S: The Diagnosis of Stupor and Coma. Ed 3. FA Davis Publishers, Philadelphia, 1980.
6. Jamieson K: Jamieson's First Notebook of Head Injury. Ed 3. Butterworth and Company Ltd, Brisbane, Calif, 1984.
7. Whyte G, Glenn M: The care and rehabilitation of the patient in a persistent vegetative state. Head Trauma Rehabilitation 1986;1:39-53.
8. Rueler JB: Hypothermia: Pathophysiology, clinical settings, and management. Ann Intern Med 1978;61:565.
9. Bauzarth: Effects of temperature upon craniocerebral trauma. JAMA 1999:135, 1976.
10. Weiss G, Feeney D, Caveness W, et al: Prognostic factors for the occurrence of post-traumatic epilepsy. Arch Neurol 1983;40:7-10.
11. Levin HS, Benton L, Guilssman RG: Neurobehavioral Consequences of Closed Head Injury. Oxford University Press Inc, New York, 1982.
12. Jeannett B: Epilepsy after Non-Missile Head Injuries. Ed 2. Heinemann, London, 1975.
13. Cuneo RA, Carrona JS: The neurological complications of hypertension. Med Clin North Am 1977;61:565.
14. Rappaport M: Survey of attitudes toward pharmacological prophylaxis of post-traumatic epilepsy. J Neurosurg 1973;38:159.
15. Williams D: EEG in traumatic epilepsy. J Neurol Neurosurg, Psychol 1944;7:103.
16. Weiss G, Caveness W: Prognostic factors in the persistence of post-traumatic epilepsy. J Neurosurg 1972;37:164-169.
17. Jeannett B: Post-traumatic epilepsy. In Rosenthal M, Griffth ER, Bond MC, et al: Rehabilitation of the Head Injured Adult. FA Davis Publishers, Philadelphia, 1983.
18. Miller JD: Volume and pressure in the craniospinal axis. Clin Neurosurg 1975;22:76.
19. Patter J: The Practical Management of Head Injury. Ed 3. Year Book Medical Publishers, Inc, Chicago, Ill, 1974.
20. Gilden J: Presentation on Pediatric Neurologic Crisis. Seventh Annual Pediatric Conference, Hamot Medical Center, Erie, Penn, September, 1986.
21. Raper AH, O'Rourke D, Kennedy S: Head position, intracranial pressure, and compliance. Neurology 1982;32:1288-1291.
22. Schneider RN, Gascch IH, Taren JA, et al: Blood vessel trauma following head and neck injuries. Clin Neurosurg 1972;19:312.
23. Bakay L, Glasauer F: Head Injury. Little, Brown Publishers, Boston, Mass, 1980.
24. Ferry DS Jr, Kenper LG: False aneurysm secondary to penetration of the brain through orbitofacial wounds. J Neurosurg 1972;36:503.
25. Clifton GL, Robertson OS, Kyper K, et al: Cardiovascular response to severe head injury. J Neurosurg 1983;59:447.
26. Braon B, Savitz MH, Elwyn DH, et al: Cerebral edema unresponsive to conventional therapy in neurosurgical patients with unsuspected nutritional failure. Crit Care Med 1973;1:125.
27. Gadissiez P, Ward JD, Young H, et al: Nutrition and the Neurosurgical Patient. J Neurosurg 1984;60:219.

28. Dempsey DT, Gunter P, Muller JL, et al: Energy expenditure in acute trauma to the head with and without barbituate therapy. Surg Gyn Obstet 1985;160:128.
29. Kaln R: Metabolic consequences of head injury. Direct in Crit Care 1985;4:1.
30. Clifton GL, et al: The metabolic response to severe head injury. J Neurosurg 1984;60:687.
31. Kudsh KA, Stone JM, Sheldon GF: Nutrition in trauma and burns. Surg Clin North Am 1982;62:183.
32. Perrin JC: Head Injury. In Molnar GE (Ed): Pediatric Rehabilitation. Williams & Wilkins Co, Baltimore, 1985, pp 207-232.
33. Jaffe MB, Mastrilli JP, Molitor CB, et al: Intervention for motor disorders. In Jlisaker M (Ed): Head Injury Rehabilitaton, Children and Adolescents. College Hill Press, San Diego, Calif, 1985.
34. Garland DE, Keenan MA: Orthopedic strategies in the management of brain injured adults. Clin Orthop 1978;131(pt 2):111-121.
35. Garland DE: Orthopedic Management of the Head Injured Adult. Reprint from the National Head Injury Foundation, Framingham, Mass, 1983.
36. Hoffer MM, Garrett A, Brink J: The orthopedic management of brain injured children. J Bone Joint Surg 1971;53-A:567-577.
37. Garland DE, Rothi B, Waters RL: Femoral fractures in head injured adults. Clin Orthop 1982;166:219-225.
38. Glenn JN, Miner ME, Peltier LJ: The treatment of fractures of the femur in patients with head injuries. J Trauma 1973;13:95-96.
39. Bellamy R, Bower TD: Management of skeletal trauma in the patient with head injury. J Trauma 1974;14(12):1021-1028.
40. Rimel RW, Jane JA: Characteristics of the head injured patient. In Rosenthal M, Griffith ER, Bond MR, et al (Eds): Rehabilitation of the Head Injured Adult. FA Davis Co, Philadelphia, 1983.
41. Berrol S: Medical assessment. In Rosenthal M, Griffith ER, Bond MR, et al (Eds): Rehabilitation of the Head Injured Adult. FA Davis Co, Philadelphia, 1983.
42. Garland DE, Bailey S: Undetected injuries in head injured adults. Clin Orthop 1981;155:162-165.
43. Rhoades ME, Garland DE: Orthopedic prognosis of brain injured adults. Clin Orthop 1978;131(pt 1):104-110.
44. Garland DE, Dowling V: Forearm Fractures in the Head Injured Adult. Clin Orthop 1983;176:190-196.
45. Garland DE, Tober L: Fractures of the tibial draphysis in adults with head injuries. Clin Orthop 1980;150:198-202.
46. Gibson JM: Multiple injuries: The management of the patient with a fractured femur and a head injury. J Bone Joint Surg 1960;42-B:425-431.
47. Garland DE, O'Hollaren RM: Fractures and dislocations about the elbow in the head injured adult. Clin Orthop 1982;168:38-41.
48. Robert PH: Heterotopic ossification complicating paralysis of intracranial origin. J Bone Joint Surg 1968;50-B:70-77.
49. Rosin AJ: Ectopic calcification around joints of paralyzed limbs in hemiplegia, diffuse brain damage, and other neurological diseases. Ann Rheum Dis 1975;34:499-505.
50. Garland DE, Razza BE, Waters RL: Forceful joint manipulation in head injured adults with heterotopic ossification. Clin Orthop 1982;169:133-138.

51. Wharton GN: Heterotopic ossification. Clin Orthop 1975;112(October):142-149.
52. Sazbon L, Najenson T, Tartakovsky M, et al: Widespread periarticular new bone formation in long term comatose patients. J Bone Joint Surg 1981;63-B:120-125.
53. Rogers CR: Presentation at the Tenth Annual Head Injury Conference. Medical College of Virginia, Williamsburg, Va, 1986.
54. Garland DE, Blum CE, Waters RL: Periarticular heterotopic ossification in head injured adults. J Bone Joint Surg 1980;62-A:1143-1146.
55. Wharton GW, Morgan TH: Ankylosis in the Paralyzed Patient. J Bone Joint Surg 1970;52-A:105-112.
56. Spielman G, Gennarelli TA, Rogers CR: Disodium etidronate: Its role in preventing heterotopic ossification. Arch Phys Med Rehabil 1983;64:539-542.
57. Wharton GW: Heterotopic ossification. Clin Orthop 1975;112:142-149.
58. Macek C: Aberrant ossification halted after head trauma. JAMA 1983;249(8):993.
59. Freed JH, Hahn H, Menter R, et al: Paraplegia 1982;20(4):208-216.
60. Norwich Eaton Pharmaceuticals, Inc. Brochure regarding uses of Didronel®. Norwich, NY, 1985.
61. Garland DE, Alday B, Venos KG, et al: Diphosphonate treatment for heterotopic ossification in spinal cord injury patients. Clin Orthop 1983;176:197-200.
62. Salter RB: Textbook of Disorders and Injuries of the Musculoskeletal System. Williams & Wilkins Co, Baltimore, 1970.
63. Adamovich B, Henderson J, Auerbach S: Cognitive Rehabilitation of Closed Head Injured Patients: A Dynamic Approach. College Hill Press, San Diego, 1985.
64. Benton A: Behavioral consequences of closed head injury. Published in Central Nervous System Trauma Research Status Report. National Institute of Neurological and Communicative Disorders and Stroke, Bethesda, Md, 1979.
65. Hagen C: Language disorders in head trauma. In Holland A (Ed): Language Disorders in Adults. College Hill Press, San Diego, 1984.
66. Caveness WF: Introduction to Head Injuries. In Walker E, Caveness W, Stichley MS (Eds): The Late Effects of Head Injury. Charles C Thomas Publisher, Springfield, Ill, 1969.
67. Benton A: Psychologic testing. In Baker AB, Baker LH (Eds): Clinical Neurology. Harper & Row Publishers Inc, New York, NY, 1974.
68. Benton A: Psychological tests for brain damage. In Freedman AM, Kaplan HI, Sadock BJ (Eds): Comprehensive Textbook of Psychiatry. Ed 2. Williams & Wilkins Co, Baltimore, 1975.
69. Ylvisaker M, Szekeres SF: Management of the patient with closed head injury. In Chapey R (Ed): Language Intervention Strategies in Adult Aphasia. Ed 2. Williams & Wilkins Co, Baltimore, 1986.
70. Wilson B, Moffat N: Clinical Management of Memory Problems. Aspen Systems Corp, Rockville, Md, 1984.
71. Rosenthal M: Behavioral sequelae. In Rosenthal M, Griffith ER, Bond MR (Eds): Rehabilitation of the Head Injured Adult. FA Davis Company, Philadelphia, 1983.
72. Dikmen S, McLean AJ, Temkin N: Neuropsychological outcome at one month post injury. Arch Phys Med Rehabil 1986;67:507.
73. Price JR: Promoting sexual wellness in head injured patients. Rehabilitation Nursing 1985;10:12-13.
74. Fryn J: Social Aspects of Traumatic Brain Injury. Presentation at the 4th Annual National Head Injury Association Conference, Boston, Mass, 1985.

75. Bishop B: Spasticity: Its physiology and management. (Pt 2) Current Concepts Concepts. Phys Ther 1977;57(pt2).
76. Griffith ER: Types of disabilities. In Rosenthal M, Griffith ER, Bond MR, et al (Eds): Rehabilitation of the Head Injured Adult. FA Davis Co, Philadelphia, 1983.
77. Griffith ER: Spasticity. In Rosenthal M, Griffith ER, Bond MR, et al (Eds): Rehabilitation of the Head Injured Adult. FA Davis Co, Philadelphia, 1983.
78. Kabat H: Proprioceptive facilitation in therapeutic exercise. In Licht S (Ed): Therapeutic Exercise. Ed 2. Waverly Press Inc, Baltimore, 1965, pp 327- 343.
79. Bishop B: Spasticity: Its physiology and management.(Pt 1): Neurophysiology of spasticity: Classical concepts. Phys Ther 1977;57:371-376.
80. Bishop B: Spasticity: Its physiology and management. (Pt 4): Current and projected treatment procedures for spasticity. Phys Ther 1977;57:397-402.
81. Caronne JJ: The neurologic evaluation. In Rosenthal M, Griffith ER, Bond MD, et al (Eds): Rehabilitation of the Head Injured Adult. FA Davis Publishers, Philadelphia, 1983.
82. Bobath B: Adult Hemiplegia: Evaluation and Treatment. (Ed 2). William Heinemann Medical Books Ltd, London, 1978.
83. Bobath K, Bobath B: Cerebral palsy. In Physical Therapy Services in the Developmental Disabilities. Charles C Thomas Publisher, Springfield, Ill, 1972.
84. Charness A: Stroke/Head Injury: A Guide to Functional Outcomes in Physical Therapy Management. Aspen Systems Corp, Rockville, Md, 1986.
85. Unpublished lecture notes, Sargent College of Allied Health Professions, Boston, Mass, February 1979.
86. Harris FA: Muscle strength receptor hypersensitivity in spasticity. Inappropriception. (Pt 3). Am J Phys Med 1978;57(1):16-28.
87. Carr JH, Sheperd RB: Physiotherapy in disorders of the brain. Heinemann Medical Books Ltd, London, 1980.
88. Harris FA: Correction of muscle imbalance in spasticity. Inapproprioception. (Pt 4). Am J Phys Med 1978;57(3):123-138.
89. Halpern D: Therapeutic exercise for cerebral palsy. In Basmajian JV (Ed): Therapeutic Exercise. (Ed 4). Williams & Wilkins Co, Baltimore, Md, 1984.
90. Sahrmann SA, Norton BJ, Bomze HA, et al: Influence of the site of lesion and muscle length on spasticity in man. Phys Ther 1974;54(12):1290-1297.
91. Bishop B: Spasticity: Its physiology and management. (Pt 4): Identifying and assessing the mechanisms underlying. Phys Ther 1977;57:385-397.
92. Babath B: Abnormal Posture Reflex Activity Caused by Brain Lesions. Ed 3. Aspen Systems Corp, Rockville, Md, 1985.
93. Brunnstrom S: Movement Therapy in Hemiplegia: A Neurophysiological Approach. Harper & Row Publishers Inc, Hagerstown, Md, 1970.
94. Class handout. April 1985. Based on Gans B: The international symposium of the traumatically brain injured child and adult. Tufts New England Medical Center, October 1981.
95. Norton BJ, Bomze HA, Chaplin H Jr: An approach to the objective measurement of spasticity. Phys Ther 1972;52(1):15-23.
96. Glenn MB: Update on pharmacology: Antispasticity medications in the patient with traumatic brain injury. J Head Trauma Rehabil 1986;1(2):71-72.
97. Glenn MB: Update on pharmacology: Nerve blocks in the treatment of spasticity. J Head Trauma Rehabil 1986;1(3):72-74.

98. Garland DE, Lucie RS, Waters RL: Current uses of open phenol nerve block for adult acquired spasticity. Clin Orthop 1982;165:217-222.

99. Braun RM, Hoffer MM, Mooney V, et al: Phenol nerve block in the treatment of acquired spastic hemiplegia in the upper limb. J Bone Joint Surg 1973;55-A:580-585.

100. Wainapel SF, Hargney D, Labib K: Spastic hemiplegia in quadriplegic patient: treatment with phenol nerve block. Arch Phys Med Rehabil 1984;65:786-787.

101. Garland DE, Lilling M, Keenan MD: Percutaneous phenol blocks to motor points of spastic forearm muscles in head injured adults. Arch Phys Med Rehabil 1984; 65:243-245.

102. Lecture notes. Sargent College of Allied Health Professions (January, 1979).

103. Harris FA: Multiple loop modulation of motor outflow: A physiological basis for facilitation techniques. Phys Ther 1971;51:391-397.

104. Sullivan PE, Markos PD, Minor MA: An Integrated Approach to Therapeutic Exercise: Theory and Clinical Application. Reston Publishing Co Inc, Reston, Va, 1982.

105. Stockmeyer SA: An interpretation of the approach of rood to the treatment of neuromuscular dysfunction. Am J Phys Med 1966;46:950-956.

106. Harris FA: Facilitation techniques and technological adjuncts in therapeutic exercise. In Basmajian JV (Ed): Therapeutic Exercise. (Ed 4). Williams & Wilkins Co, Baltimore, 1984.

107. Malovin F, Simard T: Vibration influence on control of single motor unit activity. Arch Phys Med Rehabil 1978;59:144-147.

108. Johnston RM, Bishop B, Coffey GH: Mechanical vibration of skeletal muscles. Phys Ther 1970;50:499-505.

109. Bishop B: Vibratory stimulation.(Pt 1): Neurophysiology of motor responses evoked by vibratory stimulation. Phys Ther 1974;54:1273-1281.

110. Bishop B: Vibratory stimulation.(Pt 2): Vibratory stimulation as an evaluation tool. Phys Ther 1975;55:28-34.

111. Bishop B: Vibratory stimulation. (Pt 3): Possible applications of vibration in treatment of motor dysfunctions. Phys Ther 1975;55:139-143.

112. Olson JE, Stravino VD: A review of cyrotherapy. Phys Ther 1972;52:840-853.

113. Voss DE: Proprioceptive neuromuscular facilitation. Am J Phys Med 1966;46:838-898.

114. Benton LA, Baker LL, Bowman BR: Functional Electrical Stimulation: A Practical Guide. (Ed 2). The Professional Staff Association of the Rancho Los Amigos Hospital, Inc, Downey, Calif, 1981.

115. DeBacher G: Biofeedback in spasticity control. In Basmajian JV (Ed): Biofeedback Principles and Practice for Clinicians. (Ed 2). Williams & Wilkins Co, Baltimore, 1982.

116. Kelly JL, Baker MP, Wolf SL: Procedures for EMG biofeedback training in involved upper extremities of hemiplegic patients. Phys Ther 1979;59:1500-1507.

117. Carr JH, Shepherd RB: Physiotherapy in Disorders of the Brain. William Heinemann Medical Books Ltd, London, 1980.

118. Miller JD: Early evaluation and management. In Rosenthal M, Griffith E, Bond MR, et al (Eds): Rehabilitation of the Head Injured Adult. FA Davis Co, Philadelphia, 1983.

119. Fahn S, Jankovic J: Practical management of dystonia. Neurologic Clinics: Symposium on Movement Disorders. 1984;2:555-569.
120. Russell Sage College, unpublished class notes. Ithaca, NY, April 10, 1985.

Chapter 4

ASSESSMENT FOR STATUS OF INJURY

Assessment of the head injured patient must take into consideration a multiplicity of processes and disciplines. It is necessary to assess the severity and location of the primary injury, along with an accurate evaluation of the patient's level of consciousness and cognitive functioning in relation to his level of motor and language functioning.

This process begins with diagnostic medical procedures and continues on with clinical evaluations by members of the therapy and medical staffs through assessment of support systems and involvement of significant others. It is in pooling all of this available data that we are able to, at least in general, prognosticate the patient's potential for recovery. From a neurological basis, intact brain reflexes 24 hours post injury are a significant factor in determining the recovery of the head injured patient.[1,2] These signs would include:[1]

1. Eye opening;
2. Pupillary activity;
3. Spontaneous eye movement;
4. Intact oculo-vestibular reflexes; and
5. Appropriate motor responses.

Neurological signs indicating a poor prognosis would include:

1. Nonreactive pupils;
2. Absent oculo-vestibular reflexes;
3. Severe extension patterns, or no motor response; and
4. Increased intracranial pressure.

Age has also been noted to be a significant factor in the prognosis of

Table 4-1. Factors Contributing to Severity of Head Injury.

	Mild	Moderate	Severe
Loss of Consciousness	Brief—usually < 60 minutes.	Loss of consciousness <four to six hours.	Prolonged loss of consciousness >6 hours.
Neurological changes	No obvious changes.	Abnormal neurochanges. Decreased response to stimulation. Localized only. Unequal pupils.	Abnormal neurologic signs, i.e., non-resp. pupils. Papilledema, no response to stim.
Other	Brief, often temporary retrograde amnesia.	Edema and contusion on CT scan findings.	Edema, cerebral contusion and laceration on CT.

recovery.[3] With each additional decade, age has an adverse effect. Statistically, the patient with the best prognosis for recovery is in the under 20 age group.[2]

In this chapter on the assessment of the head injured patient, the many evaluation processes available to the therapist will be discussed. Included will be diagnostic and clinical evaluations, along with a multidisciplinary evaluation which will allow for eventual interdisciplinary treatment.

Head injury is classified on the basis of type of injury to the skull, although prognosis for recovery depends primarily upon the nature and severity of damage to the brain.

A closed head injury is one in which there is either no injury to the skull, or where skull injury is limited to simple nondisplaced fracture. An open injury is usually one in which skull fragments penetrate brain tissue, such as in a severe depressed skull fracture or projectile penetration.

The severity of head injury is classified as mild, moderate, or severe (Table 4-1), based on neurological function in the first six to 24 hours.

Prediction of outcome is difficult. At best, what we have attempted to do in this chapter is to point out to the therapist how best to assess the patient's potential for rehabilitative progress based on the interrelationship of diagnostic studies and the clinical evaluation.

Diagnostic Studies

Computerized Tomography

The diagnosis and management of the head injured patient has improved dramatically since the inception of Computerized Tomography (CT). The development of CT scanning allows the direct visualization of intracranial structures. Studies show it to be a reliable diagnostic tool with an error factor of only about 3.5 percent.[4] It has become an invaluable aid in the differential diagnosis of the comatose patient. CT scan should be done as soon as possible after admission to the Emergency Room or Trauma Center. The CT will aid in locating the site of acute hemorrhages, missile tracts, epidural or subdural hematomas, along with any shift of midline structures. It will also show any shift in volume of the ventricular system.

Sequential scanning over the first two weeks post-injury aides in determining resolution of initial findings, along with the diagnosis of ongoing changes, such as increasing ventricular volume (normally evident within the first two weeks[5,6]) or new lesions. New lesions seen on a scan are often surgically treatable if done immediately.

Recent studies have been done to determine the use of CT scan to aid in prognosticating rehabilitation outcome.[7] Among the findings of Rao and associates[8] was that patients with normal CT scans were independent in all areas, while patients with bilateral lesions were dependent in all levels initially. By discharge, half of the patients had gained independence in daily living activities, while less than 15 percent achieved independence in basic intellectual skills.

Timming and associates[7] found patients with the best outcome had normal CT scans and small ventricles. Patients with enlarged ventricles had the worst outcome.[7]

While the CT scan cannot definitively predict to the therapist a patient's outcome, it does give detailed information on the severity of the injury. This, in addition to pinpointing the location of the lesion(s), can aid in establishing an initial therapy program.

Nuclear Magnetic Resonance Imaging

Nuclear Magnetic Resonance Imaging (NMRI), where available, is proving to be a tremendous diagnostic aid in the treatment of head injuries. With NMRI, magnetic radio waves, as opposed to ionizing radiation, are used to visualize cerebral lesions.[8] These radio waves, when introduced at a specific frequency, are absorbed and then re-emitted at the same frequency.[9] These re-emitted waves are then used to produce an image.

This procedure has several advantages over the more widely used CT scan. According to Davis and associates,[10] these include:

1. Better soft tissue contrast. The delineation between grey and white matter is much clearer;
2. Major blood vessels can be identified without the need for contrast media; and

3. The procedure provides better imaging of the posterior fossa.

Weinstein feels that the major drawback of NMRI is its inability to detect cortical bone and other calcification.[9] However, this appears to be only a minor problem in the use of NMRI with head injured patients, since if the cortical bone is destroyed, NMRI can detect the replacing tissue.

The potential risks of NMRI include radio frequency field exposure, varying magnetic fields, and associated risks of electrical current induction.[9] To date, no reports of such injuries have been reported in the literature. Despite the advantages of NMRI, the one major drawback with its use at this time is the inability to keep the patient on monitoring or support systems while in the imaging scanner.

Electrodiagnostics

Two types of electrodiagnostics frequently used with head injured patients are the electroencephalogram and multimodality evoked potentials. These particular studies, while not always prognostic in nature, aid the therapist in locating the focus of injury and in planning effective models of treatment.

Electroencephalography

While electroencephalography (EEG) has little use in predicting outcome in a patient with an acute head injury, it does graph manifestation of cerebral function.[11] Sharp and spike wave formation may arise from areas of focal brain damage[14] or potential epileptogenesis, while a deleted focus is often indicative of a structural lesion.[11] On occasion, however, a patient who has sustained a brainstem infarction will maintain normal alpha activity.[12] Sometimes called "alpha coma," this patient does not respond to any external stimuli as would a noncomatose patient. The prognosis for a patient in "alpha coma" is highly guarded.

Probably the most important use of the EEG in head injury is in the evaluation of post-traumatic epilepsy. EEG changes in patients exhibiting early post-traumatic seizure activity include suppression of normal frequencies and bursts of high voltage slow waves.[13]

Unfortunately, the EEG cannot be used as a diagnostic tool in predicting which patients are at risk for developing later post-traumatic epilepsy. Patients who develop late epilepsy tend to have abnormal EEGs more often than those without epilepsy. Abnormalities in the EEG are usually a reflection of damage to the brain sustained at the time of injury.[14]

Evoked Responses

Evoked responses are used to more specifically designate the responses of sensory pathways to sensory or electrical stimulation. They may be used to assess peripheral sensory function, to evaluate the functional integrity of sensory projection pathways in the central nervous system, or both.[13] The three systems generally tested are visual, auditory, and somatosensory.

Greenburg and associates[15] found evoked responses a powerful tool for making functional measurements and estimating prognosis. Abnormal multimodality evoked responses recorded accurately, consistently defined dysfunctions of visual, auditory, and motor systems in comatose patients, and were considered more effective than the clinical neurological examination in predicting residual neurologic deficits.[5]

Visual Evoked Response. Visual evoked responses (VER) measure the electrophysiologic responses of the retina and optic pathways to appropriate stimulation.[11] Cerebral VERs are the responses of cortical areas to visual stimulation.[11]

Several variations of visual stimuli may be used, but the cerebral flash evoked study appears to be best suited for the head injured patient, as the patient may not be able to reliably fixate on a pattern of stimulation.

Brainstem Auditory Evoked Responses. Brainstem Auditory Evoked Responses (BAER) detect and approximately localize dysfunctions of the auditory projection pathways.[11] The BAER provides information on the response of the auditory nerve, brain stem, and higher subcortical levels to acoustic stimuli.

Somatosensory Evoked Response. Somatosensory evoked responses (SERs) show early electrophysiologic response of the somatosensory pathways to appropriate stimulation.

Evoked potentials can be a tremendous aid to the therapist in determining an appropriate course of therapeutic action, especially in the patient who is minimally responsive. The therapist is able to determine which sensory pathways are most sensitive to stimulation, thereby allowing a therapeutic regime to be tailored to the patient. Serial evoked responses are done over a period of time and can be helpful in mapping out changes in the patient's neurologic status. It is important to note that clinical recovery often lags behind what is predicted in the evoked response, suggesting that they may be capable of pinpointing recovery and need for rehabilitation earlier than can be clinically determined.

Clinical Evaluation

The clinical evaluation differs from diagnostics in that it is based on the patient's level of functioning. The areas assessed in the clinical evaluation are

Table 4-2. Flow Sheet for Use in Tracking Patient's Level of
Consciousness Based on Glasgow Coma Scale.

		Date/ Time		Notations
Eyes	Open spontaneously	4		
	Open to sound	3		
	Open to pain	2		
	No response	1		
Motor Response	Obeys verbal command	1		
	Localizes to pain	5		
	Flexion withdrawal	4		
	Decorticate posture	3		
	Decerebrate posture	2		
	No response	1		
Verbal Response	Converses appropriately	5		
	Confused	4		
	Inappropriate	3		
	Vocalizes only	2		
	No response	1		
	Total Score			

those of cognitive functioning: level of consciousness, memory function, new learning ability, and ability to interface with one's environment.

Glasgow Coma Scale (GCS)

With the publication in 1974 of the GCS,[17] therapists and others working with the head injured patient were given a standard by which to assess the patient's level of consciousness. In essence, it takes three areas of behavior or function, which are independently measured and scored to determine the patient's level of coma. The areas scored are: eye opening, motor response, and verbal performance.

A patient with a score of 8 or less on the GCS for six hours or more is considered to have a serious head injury. One of the reasons for close, accurate monitoring of a patient's Glasgow Score is to quickly and easily detect any changes in the patient's neurological status. Any decrease in score is an indication that a CT scan should be done to rule out complications such as an acute bleed or ventricular dilatation.

Table 4-2 shows an example of a flow sheet based on the GCS which could be used to monitor the patient in the acute care setting. It is important to note that anyone working with the patient may give a score on the scale at any time. It is often useful for the therapist to keep close track of the patient's score at the beginning and end of each session. This will give the therapist an ongoing record of the patient's overall change on a daily basis and his response (or lack of response) to therapy.

The initial scorings are used as a basis for determining the severity of the patient's injuries. A patient's score may range from 3 to 15. As previously mentioned, a patient who sustains a score of 8 or less for more than six hours is considered to have a severe head injury. A patient with a score of 9 to 11 would be considered moderately head injured, and one with a score of 12 or more a mild head injury. It is vital that the initial score be obtained as soon as possible after the onset — at the scene of the accident, if possible. Once the patient is admitted, the GCS is important to quantitatively describe the patient's recovery from deep coma.[17]

It is important that all staff use the scale in a consistent manner, and that the best response elicited be scored. It should be noted on the graph if there is a reason for a no response score. For example, if the patient has a trach, he will not be able to give a verbal response. In this instance, an indication such as "T" should be placed in the corresponding "no response given" space. If the patient's eyes are bilaterally swollen, sutured closed, or bandaged, this should also be noted.

When scoring motor responses, it is the ease with which they are elicited that constitutes the criteria for best response. When giving the patient a command, it should be kept simple, such as "move your leg." Do not ask a patient to squeeze your hand, as placing your hand or other object in the patient's palm may elicit a reflexive grasp, which does not constitute following a command.

If the patient does not respond to a command, then an attempt should be made to elicit a response to pain. It is the type or quality of his reaction which constitutes the scoring criteria. If the patient moves a limb when a stimulus is applied to more than one point, he is localizing. If he withdraws from pain rapidly, he is showing a normal flexion withdrawal. However, if application of a painful stimulus creates a decorticate or decerebrate posture, these are abnormal responses. In the patient who exhibits no reaction to painful stimuli, it is important to rule out the possibility of spinal cord injury. Any difference in reaction between limbs should be carefully noted, as this may be indicative of a specific focal injury.

In differentiating among the verbal responses, the patient who converses appropriately will show an awareness of himself and his environment, while the patient who is confused will not be able to completely interface the two. The patient exhibiting inappropriate speech will not be able to sustain a conversational exchange. Only sounds or groans can be elicited from the patient

Table 4-3. Major Behaviors Exhibited by Level.

Rancho Los Amigos Scale of Cognitive Function	
Level I	No response
Level II	Generalized response
Level III	Localized response
Level IV	Confused, agitated
Level V	Confused, inappropriate
Level VI	Confused, appropriate
Level VII	Automatic, appropriate
Level VIII	Purposeful, appropriate

who is able to vocalize. Again, make note of any mechanical reason for inability to verbalize.

Spontaneous opening of the eyes indicates functioning of the ascending reticular activating system. This does not necessarily indicate the patient is aware, but does imply he is in a state of arousal (Chapter 3). The patient who opens his eyes to speech is likely responding to the stimulus of sound, not necessarily to a command to open his eyes. The therapist may wish to try different sound making objects (bell, horn, etc.) to elicit a reaction. If the patient does not respond to sound, a painful stimulus must be applied. The stimulus should not be applied to the face, as this may cause the eyes to close tightly in a protective reaction.

The patient's GCS should be monitored in the acute setting until full responsiveness is established, or until the patient is transferred to a rehabilitation unit or facility.

Rancho Los Amigos Scale of Cognitive Functioning

While the GCS gives the therapist an accurate assessment of the patient's levels of consciousness and recovery during the early acute phase, the Rancho Los Amigos Scale of Cognitive Functioning[18] behaviorally assesses the patient's cognitive abilities. Patients are rated on the Ranchos Scale by correlating behavior with orientation, attention, memory processing abilities, appropriateness, and organizational abilities.

The Ranchos Scale[18] (Table 4-3) is an eight-level progression from Level I, where the patient is nonresponsive, to Level VIII, where the patient's behavior is purposeful and appropriate. The Ranchos Scale was developed as a behavioral rating system to aid in the assessment of cognitive recovery. It should be stressed that the Ranchos Scale is an assessment of cognitive functioning and behavior *only*, not of physical functioning. It is not unusual to work with a patient who, because of the location of his or her injury has total motoric involvement, but is functioning at a high cognitive level. Conversely, a patient may be physically functional, but may be extremely confused and disoriented.

The patient's level of cognitive awareness is evaluated by observing the patient in both structured and unstructured settings. Both verbal and nonverbal activities are included. Duration and frequency of behavior is also taken into consideration when determining the patient's level of functioning. Some facilities have found the addition of a plus (+) or minus (−) following the level (or combined levels) to indicate the patient is showing behaviors consistent with more than one level or is in transition between levels.

Management approaches based on the Rancho Los Amigos Scale of Cognitive Functioning will be discussed in detail in Chapter 5.

In order for the therapist to appropriately classify the patient, we have included a brief description of behaviors exhibited at each level.

Level I. There is a complete absence of observable behavioral change to visual, auditory, or painful stimuli.

Level II. There is a generalized reflex response to painful stimuli and the patient only responds inconsistently to auditory stimuli. It should be noted that response to stimulation may be with physiological changes, i.e., increased pulse, respirations, or diaphoresis.

Level III. Here, the patient responds in a specific manner to specific stimuli. He will withdraw from painful stimuli, focus on a presented object, track in the horizontal place, turn his head toward sound, and may inconsistently respond to simple commands.

Level IV. At this level, the patient is in a state of internal, generalized confusion. He is in a heightened state of activity, but has a severely decreased ability to interact with his environment. His behavior often appears to be grossly out of proportion to the stimuli or environment. Verbalization may be present, but is often incoherent.

Level V. The Level V patient remains confused, but has the ability to demonstrate gross attention to his environment. Memory function is severely impaired with responses being inappropriate. Additionally, there is no carryover for newly learned information. He may continue to have periods of agitation, but these can usually be attributed to external stimuli.

Level VI. The Level VI patient is inconsistently oriented to time and place.

While organizational skills remain poor, the patient is capable of new learning. He will consistently follow commands, but memory function remains poor.

Level VII. There is the ability to function in an appropriate manner within a structured setting. There is also increasing carryover for new memory; however, judgment and reasoning remain problematic.

Level VIII. Within his physiological limitations, the patient is essentially independent in all areas. He is often appropriate for vocational considerations, and exhibits appropriate judgment on an independent level.

Post-traumatic Amnesia

Recent studies[14,19-24] have all shown a definite correlation between the duration of Post-Traumatic Amnesia (PTA) and cognitive recovery in the head injured patient. Studies by Russell[20] in the late 60s were among the first to use PTA to assess the severity of diffuse brain damage.

PTA is considered to be the length of time from injury until such time as conscious memory returns.[19]

The duration of PTA is believed to be directly related to the severity of injury.[14,19] A patient who sustains a period of PTA less than 60 minutes is considered to have sustained a mild head injury. One whose period of PTA lasts from one to 24 hours has a moderate injury, while the patient whose duration of PTA lasts more than one week is considered to have sustained a very serious head injury.

Miller[19] has noted that when the duration of PTA is greater than seven days, full return of neurologic function would be highly unusual.

There does appear to be some dissension among the experts as to when a patient has recovered from PTA. Jeannett[14] states it is the point in time at which the patient becomes aware of his surroundings. Gronwall and Wrigtson[23] indicate it is the number of days for a patient to be able to do serial addition tasks.

For practical purposes, we have chosen the criterion from Kameron and associates,[24] which indicates that the period of PTA is considered over when the patient is able to follow a two-step verbal command. This particular criterion precludes the one drawback pointed out by Berrol,[25] which is that most criteria require the patient's ability to speak, which is often delayed. It also indicates the patient's ability to process data and perform an activity based on previously learned tasks.

This criterion also makes assessment of the duration of PTA a practical tool for the therapist, as it is based on a combination of the patient's cognitive and functional abilities.

Therapeutic Evaluations

Occupational Therapy Evaluation

As with evaluations from other disciplines, evaluation by the occupational therapist begins with a thorough review of the medical record. Notation should be made as to the duration of coma, type and location of injury, and scores in the GCS as well as other information pertinent to the evaluation, such as additional injuries (i.e., fractures), and early abnormal posturing.

The main goals of the occupational therapy evaluation include evaluation and assessment of perceptual motor skills, upper extremity functioning, positioning, need for adaptive equipment, activities of daily living, sensory functioning, fine motor control, and eye/hand coordination. In addition, dependent on the facility's delineation of therapeutic responsibility, evaluation of feeding and swallowing skills may be performed by the occupational therapist.

Impaired perceptual motor skills will be a major limiting factor in ultimate functional outcome and are likely to remain as a permanent residual deficit to some degree. The perceptual/motor deficits as described in Chapter 3 will affect the occupational therapist's approach or the patient's response to occupational therapy interventions. For example, in the patient with a right/left discrimination deficit, he or she will need tactile input to follow simple motor commands for a given extremity. The therapist can then also incorporate strategies to improve perceptual/motor problems into her treatment program.

In the evaluation of upper extremity function, the perspective of the occupational therapist in assessing this functional use can aid the physical therapist in delineating specific causes of dysfunction. It is also important to note alterations in muscle tone, movement patterns, and passive range of motion at varying time intervals and during a variety of activities. These factors can fluctuate several times in the course of any given day.

When developing positioning procedures specific to the needs of the head injured patient, resting positions and responses to alterations in position must be frequently monitored. An assessment is then done to provide appropriate modifications.

The occupational therapy evaluation of activities of daily living and need for adaptive equipment will also give the physical therapist a picture of how the patient's physical dysfunctions are affecting his overall functional independence.

Frequently, the occupational therapy evaluation will include the patient's ability to manage his time, the amount of structure required, and his ability to interact with other patients, family, and friends. The physical therapist should not place excessive demands on the patient's orientation or memory functioning when providing therapy. The patient should be allowed to succeed, but also be stimulated and challenged. The information provided by the occupational therapist will assist the physical therapist in optimally structuring the patient's sessions.

Speech Therapy Evaluation

A speech-language pathologist assesses the complex, sequential process of communication. This evaluation consists of formal and information observation and measurement of oral motor skills which are necessary for the vegetative function of swallowing and for the secondary function of speech production. Language and cognitive abilities are assessed by the speech-language pathologist.

Speech is the actual physical activity of producing sound. Following a closed head injury, some patients have difficulty speaking due to a weakness or lack of coordination of muscle movements needed for speech and voice production. In the closed head injury patient, speech may be slurred, imprecise, unintelligible, or totally absent. The oral motor weakness may also be reflected in decreased biting, chewing, swallowing, and eating skills.

Language is comprised of two aspects, receptive and expressive. Receptive language consists of understanding spoken or written information. Expressive language is viewed as the communication of needs and wants through the verbal, gestural, or written modalities.

Language disorders occur in many variations. Specific receptive language disorders which are identified during diagnostic procedures include difficulties understanding spoken and written language, decreased auditory and visual retention span, and reduced word recognition.

Expressive language problems may be evident in naming abilities, grammar, syntax, confused verbalizations, and a reduced ability to write.

The most common problem a patient experiences following a closed head injury is a decrease in cognitive functioning or information processing. This means that a patient is experiencing difficulty with concentration, attention, orientation, memory, categorizing, sequencing, judgment, reasoning, and problem solving. When cognitive functioning is decreased, it is reflected in all areas of interaction an individual has with the environment.

Patients who demonstrate difficulty with hearing are referred to an audiologist who will assess hearing capabilities. Appropriate recommendations from the audiologist will be implemented by all treating team members.

Because of the complexity of the communication process, it is helpful for individuals working with the head injured patient to remember that speech, language, or cognitive problems may occur in isolation or may coexist. To effectively communicate with the head injured, it is best to explain ideas in a consistent manner, to allow sufficient time for the individual to process the information, and to respond verbally or with the communication system established by the speech-language pathologist.

Physical Therapy Assessment

Physical therapy evaluations should delineate the patient's abilities as well as dysfunctions. The evaluation process should be ongoing, and occur on a daily basis to assess immediate response to treatment, and at regular intervals to document progress.

The initial evaluation must provide a solid baseline to identify problems and goals, plan treatments, and compare interval changes and response to the treatment program.

The assessment must be modified for the head injured patient, taking into consideration the extent of cognitive deficits. A thorough history must be obtained from the medical record or family. It is important to note the date and type of injury, cause of injury, and length of coma, as these factors all have some predictive value in determining outcome, and will alert the therapist to some specific evaluation procedures. Medical complications as a result of the injury, subsequent surgical interventions, and premorbid medical history could affect treatment and the choice of evaluation procedures. Medications must be reviewed in light of their effect on the patient's ability to participate in the evaluation and for any effects they may have on evaluation findings.

A review of the patient's premorbid social history is helpful as the patient will most likely respond better to familiar topics of conversation. This will also provide the therapist with information to assess memory functioning.

The first step in the physical therapy assessment is to assess the patient's cognitive and behavioral status to guide appropriate selection of evaluation procedures. Does the patient respond to name call? Can he respond to indicate yes or no? Can he follow simple or complex commands?

It is also important to note the patient's status without any intervention. Does he demonstrate any awareness of the environment? Does he have any spontaneous movement and is that movement random or purposeful? What is the patient's resting position? Is he demonstrating abnormal posturing?

While assessing the low level patient (nonresponsive or minimally responsive), look for a generalized or localized response to pain, tactile stimulation, visual stimulation, and auditory stimulation. Does the patient open his eyes? Can he focus or localize to sound? Can he follow a simple, one-step command? If the response is delayed, note the length of the delay. The command must be within the patient's motoric abilities.

In the alert, responsive patient, note delay in responses, ability to follow one, two, or three step commands within motor abilities, orientation, memory, and attention span. How long can the patient attend to a task? During the evaluation session, note if the patient becomes distracted by extraneous activity. Can he complete a task? Does he perseverate on tasks or verbalizations? Are verbalizations confused? Also note if the patient becomes agitated, including stimulus and duration of agitation. Is the patient verbally abusive or physically aggressive? Can he be redirected or calmed with "time out" procedures or explanations?

A brief assessment of communication skills should include initiation of verbalization, or verbalization in response to questions. Is speech intelligible and appropriate? Does the patient communicate nonverbally with gestures, head nods, or other systems? Comment on consistency and delay time of responses.

Physical assessment must also vary according to cognitive level. Sensation cannot be assessed in the minimally responsive patient, and is unlikely to be accurately reported in the agitated or confused patient. A gross assessment of the patient's sensory status can be obtained by observing the agitated or confused patient interacting within his environment. In the mid to high level patient, a complete sensory evaluation includes light touch discrimination, sharp/dull discrimination, hot/cold discrimination, pressure, kinesthesia, and proprioception. Record whether sensations are intact, impaired, or absent.

If light touch is intact, assess tactile localization and extinction. Also note tactile hypersensitivity and patient complaints of abnormal sensation or pain. Be aware of the fact that head injured patients may frequently overreact to a stimulus, and can perceive any stimulus as pain.

Passive range of motion can be evaluated on all patients except the agitated patient. Observation of the agitated patient's spontaneous and volitional movements can alert the therapist to possible joint limitations. Determine the causes of any limitations, i.e., joint restriction, pain, abnormal muscle tone, or contracture. Passive range of motion should be evaluated in varying positions in the presence of abnormal postural reactions.

Active movement can be assessed in all patients, grossly through observation and specifically through functional muscle testing in patients who can follow commands or demonstrations. Note whether movement is isolated or in synergy, mass or advanced patterns, coordinated, etc. Evaluate for the presence of movement disorders (i.e., ataxia, tremors, athetosis). Also note speed of movement and ability to reverse antagonist. If movement occurs only with facilitation, also note the type of facilitation used.

Assessment of tone includes resistance to passive stretch and response to tapping vibration and ice. Tone should be assessed in varying positions and positions noted. Also assess tone while performing an activity. Determine what increases or decreases tone in each patient.

Reflex testing can be carried out on all patients. Note if reflexes are obligatory or if the reflex influence can be inhibited by the patient consciously (i.e., ask the patient to turn his head to the left without letting his left elbow extend). Evaluate righting and equilibrium responses.

Coordination can be observed in patients with cognitive Levels III, IV, and sometimes V. Patients who can attend to tasks and follow directions consistently (Levels V through VIII) can be evaluated for incoordination with standard test procedures, including assessing rapid alternating movements, finger to nose, finger to finger, finger dexterity, heel to shin, and foot tapping. Document speed and quality of movement. Also perform tests for Romberg's Sign in patients who are able to stand. Evaluate posture in supine, sitting, and standing as appropriate. Determine the cause of any postural deviations (e.g., spasticity) and the need for adaptive equipment.

Skin condition needs to be evaluated for integrity and potential problem areas as well as any signs of swelling, warmth, or redness, which may be indicative of thrombophlebitis or heterotopic ossification.

Gross motor control can be assessed in patients who are able to follow commands. Document stages of motor control achieved in each posture. Response to handling and movement in and out of developmental postures can be evaluated in the minimally responsive patient.

Balance should be assessed in sitting and standing, with and without upper extremity support, statically and dynamically.

Functional assessment should include transfers to and from the bed, wheelchair, mat table, floor, toilet, etc. Document the amount of physical assistance needed as well as the amount of structure and cueing. Also assess bed mobility, vertical and horizontal scooting, bridging, rolling, and the ability to edge-of-bed sit prior to transfer. Wheelchair mobility would address level surfaces, ramps, doorways, elevators, and use of accessories (brakes, removable arm rests).

Ambulatory status should note the amount of assistance required, structure, cueing on level and uneven surfaces, and stairs. Note the type of devices used, endurance, and any gait deviations. Note if deviations are correctable with verbal, tactile, or proprioceptive cueing. Does the patient demonstrate awareness of limitations and safety issues? With independently ambulatory patients, assess higher level balance and coordination abilities by observing the patient's ability to hop, jump, skip, run, perform braiding, and coordinate lower extremities while following complex directions; i.e., perform hopscotch pattern for five feet then jump over tape marks starting with the right foot and alternating jumps. Also assess the patient's ability to climb ladders and bend and straighten while moving various objects to a variety of surfaces.

Many of the evaluation procedures may not be appropriate for all cognitive levels and also may not be appropriate for all patients with varying degrees of physical impairment. Much of the evaluation report will be narrative to describe the quality of responses and quality of movement. For ease of comparison, the therapist may wish to use a checklist/graphic format to record concrete data for the initial and subsequent evaluations.

A sample evaluation format has been provided. Once this evaluation is completed, the therapist should summarize his or her findings to give an assessment of the patient's abilities/limitations, areas amenable to treatment, and prognosis for therapeutic intervention.

Examples of physical therapy evaluation forms are given in Appendices A through K.

Support Systems Evaluation

One particular area often left out when doing an assessment of the head injured patient is that of family dynamics. Often as professionals, we forget that our patient is a member of a tightly woven structure in which all members are dependent on each other.

It is important to assess early on both family structure and involvement. This assessment should include not only the nuclear family, but also extended family and significant others who will play a part in the patient's recovery and rehabilitation process.

The patient's premorbid role in the family structure, the family's previous coping skills, and their knowledge of the recovery process from head injury are all necessary in making a thorough assessment of the patient.

Studies have found that many patients do not reach their full potential, not only due to their own inability to develop adequate coping mechanisms, but also due to the failure of the family to give the patient help and support toward a full recovery.[26] Often the family is uninvolved due to fear or lack of understanding of the head injury recovery process. This should indicate to the therapist the need for intervention, emotional support, and education.

Family interaction with staff members must also be assessed to determine if family members may be avoiding or manipulating staff members. Evaluation of the kind and quality of these interactions will also assist the therapist in the development of educational experiences appropriate to the family's capabilities.

The above mentioned factors should indicate to the therapist and the treatment team the need to be acutely aware of the patient's position in the family, his relationship with family members and significant others, and the family's ability to support the patient for a prolonged period of time.

The family's role on the therapy team, ability to cope with a head injured loved one, and education will be dealt with in Chapter 5 on rehabilitation.

References

1. Bach Y-Rita P: Recovery of Function: Theoretical Considerations for Injury Rehabilitation. University Park Press, Baltimore, Md, 1980.
2. Gildchrist E, Wilkinson M: Some factors determining prognosis in young people

with severe head injury. Arch Neurol 1979;36:355-359.

3. Jeannett B, Teasdale G: Management of Head Injuries. FA Davis, Philadelphia, 1981.

4. Baker H, Campbell S, Hanson O, et al: Computer assisted tomography of head: Early evaluation. Mayo Clin Proc 1974;49:17-24.

5. Kashore P, Lippen M, Muler J: Post-traumatic hydrocephalus in patients with severe head injury. Neuroradiology 1978;16:261-265.

6. Burk J, Imleus C, Woo-Sem J: Physical recovery after severe closed head trauma in children and adults. J Pediatr 1980;97:24-27.

7. Timming R, Orrison W, Mikula J: CT and rehabilitation outcome after severe head trauma. Arch Phys Med Rehabil 1982;63:154-159.

8. Rao N, Jellinek H, Harvey R, et al: CT head scans as predictions of rehabilitation outcome. Arch Phys Med Rehabil 1984;65:1980.

9. Weinstein M: Nuclear Magnetic Resonance. Lecture from Update in Management of the Neurologic Client seminar. Cleveland Clinic, Cleveland, Ohio, 1985.

10. Davis PD, Kaufman L, Crooks LE, et al: Techniques in imaging of the brain: (Pt B). Nuclear magnetic resonance imaging. In Rosenberg RN (Ed): The Clinical Neurosciences. Churchill Livingstone Inc, New York, Edinburgh, 1984.

11. Aymone-Marsan C (Editor-in-chief): American EEG Society Guidelines in EEG and Evoked Potentials, 1986. J Clin Neurophysical 1986;3(suppl): 34-37.

12. Peilo VP: The use of the electroencephalogram in the evaluation of head trauma. N Engl J Med 1967;276:104.

13. Williams D: EEG in traumatic epilepsy. J Neurol Neurosurg Psychiatry 1944;7:103.

14. Jeannett B: Post-traumatic epilepsy. In Rosenthal M, Griffith ER, Bond MR, et al (Eds): Rehabilitation of the Head Injured Adult. FA Davis Co, Philadelphia, 1983, p 122.

15. Greenburg RP, et al: Prognostic implications of early multimodality evoked potentials in severely head injured patients. A prospective study. J Neurosurg 1981;55:227.

16. Nerolon PG, Greenburg RP: Assessment of brain function with multimodality evoked potentials. In Rosenthal M, Griffith ER, Bond MR, et al (Eds): Rehabilitation of the Head Injured Adult. FA Davis Co, Philadelphia, 1983, p 93.

17. Teasdale G, Jennett B: Assessment of coma and impaired consciousness: A practical scale. Lancet 1974;2:81-84.

18. Hagen C, Malkmus D, Durham P: Levels of cognitive functioning. In Rehabilitation of the Head Injured Adult. Comprehensive Management. Professional Staff Association of Rancho Los Amigos Hospital, Downey, Calif, 1980.

19. Miller JD: Early evaluation and management. In Rosenthal M, Griffith ER, Miller JD, et al: Rehabilitation of the Head Injured Adult. FA Davis Co, Philadelphia, 1983.

20. Russell WR: The Traumatic Amnesias. Oxford Univ Press Inc, London, 1971.

21. Brasko DN, Aughton ME: Psychological consequences of blunt head injury. Int Rehabil Med 1979;1:160.

22. Brasko DN, Aughton ME: Cognitive recovery during the first year after blunt head injury. Int Rehabil Med 1979;1:160.

23. Gronwail V, Wrighton P: Cumulative effective of concussion. Lancet 1975;2:995.

24. Kamron T, Mathis S, Zazula T: Cognitive recovery after moderate and severe head injury. In Darcy RG, Winn HR, Rimel RW, et al: Trauma of the Central Nervous System. Raven Press Pubs, New York, 1985.
25. Berrol S: Medical Assessment. In Rosenthal M, Griffith ER, Bond MR, et al (Ed): Rehabilitation of the Head Injured Adult. FA Davis Publishers, Philadelphia, 1983.
26. Epperson M: Families in crisis: Process and intervention in a critical care unit. Soc Work Health Care 1977;2:265.

Chapter 5

REHABILITATION IN
THE ACUTE CARE SETTING

As with all physical therapy treatments of neurological patients, a thorough evaluation of the head injured patient must be completed, and appropriate, goal-directed therapy devised. Treatment for neurological dysfunction should be aimed at development of autonomic homeostasis, integration of reflexes, and development of normal movement to promote skillful functional abilities.

There are a vast number of treatment approaches available to the physical therapist to achieve these general goals. There are some principles unique to each approach, but all of the approaches have many areas of overlap. Various authors have contributed to the body of knowledge available to physical therapists in the area of therapeutic exercise. Although the treatment techniques described in this chapter are not specifically referenced, an extensive bibliography is included at the end of this book. This section on treatment techniques is to assist the therapist in planning treatments that will address the cognitive and physical sequelae of head injury. Not every treatment is meant for every patient, and the therapist must very carefully evaluate each individual patient's response to each component of her therapy program. Some of the techniques discussed will be useful with patients at all cognitive levels, while others may only be appropriate with a very low or high level patient. Many problems can be present with patients of all cognitive levels.

The physical problems of the head injured patient are not entirely different from those of other patients with CNS disorders. The extent of the problems may be more severe. The treatment approaches are based on the same neurophysiological, biomechanical, and tonal influences. Modification and adjustment of activities are made to incorporate cognitive goals or to get around cognitive deficits. Tonal disorders in head injury have similarities and differences to tonal disorders in CVA, multiple sclerosis, cerebral palsy, etc. Abnormal reflexes or movement disorders in head injury are similar to abnormal reflex and movement disorders in cerebral palsy. Treatment progression is based on the same physical factors, with careful consideration of cognitive limitations. The vast number of problems each head injured patient may present with can seem overwhelming at first, but the problems can be systematically analyzed, and creative, goal-directed treatment programs devised.

In treating the head injured patient, the therapist must keep in mind that she is not treating the head injury and cannot change the extent of brain injury. The therapist is treating the sequelae of head injury: the cognitive, physical, and behavioral deficits that occur as a result of the brain injury.

Physical treatment is aimed at preventing secondary complications and "directing" motor responses returning as a result of spontaneous recovery (decreasing edema, plasticity of the CNS). Optimally, any form of treatment should be directed toward meeting several goals at once.

Therapeutic intervention with the head injured patient must begin in the acute care setting to provide optimal potential for rehabilitation.[1-6] Physical therapy can begin in the Intensive Care Unit to prevent pulmonary and musculoskeletal complications.[1,5,7,8] The Maryland Institute for Emergency Medical Services found the best approach to treatment of the acute head injured patient in the Intensive Care Unit is through the development of treatment protocols with the medical, nursing, and physical therapy staff, close interaction between staffs, staff education, and close monitoring of changes in intracranial pressure in response to positioning and treatment.[1]

Depending on the staffing pattern of the hospital, chest physical therapy may be provided by physical therapists, respiratory therapists, or both. Chest physical therapy can include positioning, percussion, vibration, suctioning, coughing, and breathing exercises.[1,5] Postural drainage may have to be temporarily discontinued with excessive increase in intracranial pressure.[1,6] The primary goal of physical therapy in the Intensive Care Unit during the acute phase is to prevent secondary complications.[1,7,8]

The Low Level Patient

The primary goals with patients demonstrating cognitive levels of I, II, and III are to increase level of arousal, increase responsiveness, and limit or prevent secondary complications. The therapist must provide stimulation as well as provide traditional therapeutic measures.

In addition to the stimulation provided during patient care, a structured program of sensory stimulation should be carried out several times per day and be provided by all disciplines working with the patient (Physical Therapy,

Occupational Therapy, Nursing, Speech Therapy, Therapeutic Recreation, and Neuropsychology), as well as by significant others. Careful documentation of responses including number of trials presented, type of stimulus, number of trials responded to, and intensity, duration, and variety of responses must be completed to assess the most appropriate channels of intervention and patient progress.

Stimulation should begin at a very basic level and progress to advanced as the patient demonstrates consistency of response to any given stimulus. Only one sensory system should be stimulated at any one time. Stimulation should not be provided continuously as this allows the system to accommodate. The therapist must allow the patient adequate time to respond to any given stimulus and note if the response is generalized or localized. The patient will be more responsive to familiar items such as known scents, family members, family pictures, tapes of family voices, sounds related to previous employment or leisure activities (i.e., fireman-alarm, teacher-school bell, baseball player-bat connecting with ball, etc.), favorite foods, etc.

Stimulation must be provided in a quiet area to allow the patient to direct his limited abilities to the presented stimulus. Extraneous stimulation should be minimized. Whenever possible, lessen or remove painful equipment, turn off the television or radio, etc. However, if the patient needs to be aroused prior to providing stimulation, uncomfortable positioning and painful stimuli preceding presentation of stimulation may be helpful; i.e., press the patient's fingernails immediately before asking the patient to look at his mother's picture, push patient off balance (fright = fight or flight response) immediately before giving a command to pick up an object.

Arousal techniques may also increase spasticity and therefore must be closely monitored. The goal of stimulation is to progress the patient to the next cognitive level as described in Chapter 4.

As the Level I patient has no observable responses to any type of stimulation, the goal of stimulation would be to evoke a generalized response to any sensory input (i.e., increased respirations, eye opening, including only reflexive responses). In the Level II patient who is already demonstrating generalized responses, the goal is to localize the response to the stimulus (i.e., turn toward the sound), and increase nonreflexive responses. The Level III patient responds to specific stimuli in a delayed and inconsistent manner, and therefore, the goal of stimulation is to increase consistency and variety of responses, and to channel responses into functional activities. Table 5-1 outlines the sensory input and desired generalized and localized responses.

Bed positioning should be devised to promote pulmonary toilet, prevent skin breakdown, inhibit abnormal reflexes, prevent contractures, and encourage interaction with the environment. To maintain skin integrity, the patient should be repositioned every two hours. Useful positions include supine prone, sidelying, 45 degrees from supine, and 45 degrees from prone. Varying these

Table 5-1. Stimulation.

System	Stimuli	Desired Response
Visual	1. Light 2. Faces 3. Objects	Focusing Tracking
Auditory	1. Loud sounds—bells, clapping 2. Music 3. Voice—greetings, explanations of all procedures.	Eye opening, change in muscle tone or respirations, localizing toward sound or away from sound. Follow one step commands.
Olfactory	Various scents (pleasant and noxious)	Eye opening, change in muscle tone or respirations, grimacing, move toward or away from stimulus.
Tactile	Various textures, temperatures, pressures (pleasant and noxious)	Eye opening, change in muscle tone or respirations, moving stimulated part toward or away from stimulus.
Kinesthetic	Movement	Eye opening, change in muscle tone or respirations, look at part being moved, withdraw extremity being moved, attempt to reposition self, assist with desired movement.

positions will not only prevent pressure on bony prominences, but also provide postural drainage of the uppermost portions of the lungs. Visually stimulating items should be strategically placed to be within the patient's visual field in each position. Prevention of contractures can be achieved through specific modifications of each of these positions to affect alterations in muscle tone, abnormal posturing, and pathological reflexes.

To minimize excessive extensor tone in the supine position, modifications are directed toward decreasing the influence of decerebrate or decorticate posturing and tonic neck and labyrinthine reflexes. The bed can be elevated at the headboard and footboard to increase trunk, hip, and knee flexion. A foam wedge, pillow, or towel roll can be placed under the knees to position the hips and knees in flexion while providing a soft surface to possibly facilitate the hamstrings.

Sandbags or cervical supports can be utilized to maintain the head and neck in a neutral midline position to eliminate the effect of the asymmetrical tonic neck reflex, symmetrical tonic neck reflex, and symmetrical tonic labyrinthine

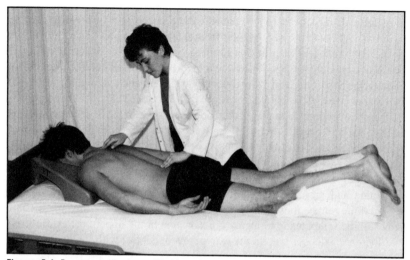

Figure 5-1. Prone positioning with hips abducted and knees flexed. The therapist is applying slow stroking down the posterior primary rami for generalized inhibition of tone. Photos taken by Michael Plasha, courtesy of Lake Erie Institute of Rehabilitation.

reflex. In the patient who demonstrates decerebrate posturing unilaterally, positioning could make use of the influence of the asymmetrical tonic neck reflex by positioning the head rotated toward the affected side to encourage flexor tone in the extended extremities.

In the presence of decorticate positioning (upper extremities flexed, lower extremities extended), positioning the neck in some extension could utilize the influence of the symmetrical tonic neck reflex to encourage extensor tone in the upper extremities and flexor tone in the lower extremities. Firm wedges and bivalved casts with spreader bars can decrease adductor spasticity, maintain hips in abduction, and break up a spastic extensor pattern in the lower extremities. Soft pillows or foam wedges should not be used, as they may facilitate increased adductor spasticity. Air splints may be beneficial to decrease adductor and plantarflexor tone and are available in long leg, short leg, and cylinder versions for the lower extremities. Short leg casts or bivalves, molded ankle-foot orthoses, and high-top sneakers can maintain neutral position and inhibit tone in the plantar flexors. Towel rolls can be utilized to encourage pelvic or scapula protraction.

The prone position is especially useful for preventing hip flexor contractures and draining the posterior segments of the lungs. This position may be contraindicated in the very early stages and will require continuous close monitoring. A prone pillow with an opening to accommodate the face and tracheostomy assists in maintaining an open airway. Prone encourages flexor tone via the symmetrical tonic neck reflex, and therefore is the best position to remove equipment (bivalved casts, splints) from the feet. A pillow placed under the lower legs increases knee flexion to break up the extensor pattern. The upper extremities should be positioned down by the patient's side in the presence of decorticate posturing, and in shoulder flexion and abduction, and elbow flexion in the presence of decerebrate posturing. In the presence of unilateral posturing, the head can be rotated to utilize the opposing affects of the asymmetrical tonic neck reflex and provide prolonged passive stretch to neck musculature. Towel rolls can be utilized to promote scapula or pelvic retraction. A wedge can still be useful to decrease adductor tone (Figure 5-1).

Positioning in sidelying is based on the same neurophysiological principles as supine and prone. In sidelying, the influence of the asymmetrical tonic labyrinthine reflex must be overcome or utilized. The asymmetrical tonic labyrinthine reflex tends to increase flexor tone in the uppermost extremities, and increase extensor tone in the extremities in contact with the bed.

Table 5-2. Tonal Changes Associated with Tonic Reflexes.

Reflex	Stimulus	Response
Asymmetrical tonic neck reflex	Head rotation	Increased extensor tone in extremities on chin side Increased flexor tone in extremities on skull side
Symmetrical tonic neck reflex	1. Head flexion 2. Head extension	Increased flexor tone in upper extremities Increased extensor tone in lower extremities Increased extensor tone in upper extremities Increased flexor tone in lower extremities
Asymmetrical tonic labyrinthine reflex	Sidelying	Increased flexor tone in uppermost extremities Increased extensor tone in lowermost extremities (In contact with supporting surface)
Symmetrical tonic labyrinthine reflex	1. Head extension in supine 2. Head flexion in prone	Increased extensor tone throughout all extremities Increased flexor tone throughout all extremities

Although excessive flexor tone is less commonly seen after head injury, devising an appropriate positioning program is based on the same general principles.

In the presence of pathological primitive reflexes, positioning may need to be altered out of reflex postures as opposed to utilizing the influence of these reflexes (Table 5-2).

The patient should get out of bed as soon as possible to prevent osteoporosis by weight bearing through the spine, provide the feeling of upright positioning, loosen secretions from posterior walls of the lungs, provide visual stimulation and an increased ability to interact with the environment, and to provide stress to the cardiovascular system. The sitting position can also be used to inhibit pathological tonic reflexes. With close monitoring, positioning the patient out of bed should ideally begin in the Intensive Care Unit. Sitting alleviates the pressure to the sacrum, heels, and bony prominences, and limits cardiovascular changes of decreased blood flow to the extremities and decreased systolic blood

Table 5-3. Wheelchair Positioning Options (with Predominantly Extensor Tone).

Pelvis:	Backrest at 75 degrees with hard wedge to provide support (no pull of gravity) and maintain hip and trunk flexion at 90 degrees.
Spine:	Lumbar roll to maintain normal lordosis. Seat belt across pelvis. Scoliosis pads or Vac-Pacs® to maintain upper trunk alignment. Upper trunk strap and/or laptray.
Head:	Extended head support. Options: Head well Pillow Theraband® Slings/outrigger Collar (Philadelphia, AOA, SOMI) Cast
Lower Extremities:	Cushion or padding to rotate pressure. Rolls along thighs to prevent external rotation. Theraband to facilitate abduction and prevent ER. AB wedge (hard) to prevent adduction. Knees at 90 degrees. Firm surface for gastrocsoleus, calf pad. Ankle straps to prevent knee extension and maintain contact (hard) with feet. Wedges on foot pedals to increase dorsiflexion.

pressure.[9] The influence of tonic reflexes is lessened in the sitting position,[10] and righting reactions can be developed. Sitting stimulates the visual, kinesthetic, and vestibular systems. Wheelchair positioning should follow the same principles of bed positioning. Examples of possible modifications for head, trunk, and extremity alignment have been provided for patients demonstrating predominantly extensor tone in Table 5-3.

While the patient must remain in the ICU, acute surgical, or neuro unit, treatment does not have to be limited to passive range of motion exercises, positioning, and sensory stimulation. Handling techniques to promote righting and equilibrium reactions can be initiated at the bedside. Mat activities can begin in bed to decrease abnormal muscle tone and promote active movement. Activities such as slow rocking in bilateral sidelying can be used to decrease tone and provide vestibular and tactile stimulation. Rhythmic initiation can be utilized to promote active movement. Once a slight decrease in trunk rigidity is obtained, pelvic and scapular rotation can be initiated segmentally and progressed to counter-rotation. The upper extremities can be mobilized into a thrusting or diagonal pattern. The effect of gravity will be eliminated, and the patient may assist with the movement. The unaware patient will be receiving kinesthetic and proprioceptive stimulation.

Simple explanations should be given to the patient before initiating any activity to prevent fright and a subsequent increase in tone. Therapists should repeat what is being carried out to maintain arousal and vary tone of voice and timing to provide further stimulation. If the patient is demonstrating any movements, quick stretch and resistance should be added to facilitate even more movement. These bed activities will also stimulate loosening of pulmonary secretions.

Edge of bed sitting can be utilized to promote equilibrium and balance reactions, allow weight bearing on upper extremities to normalize tone, give the patient a feeling of the upright position, and work on facilitation of head and trunk control. This posture also allows weight bearing through the spine to prevent disuse osteoporosis. The therapist can sit behind the patient, use her thighs to stabilize at the pelvis, use her arms to control upper trunk, and use her hands to control head position. The therapist can then manipulate the patient's body by her movements. Rotational activities can be utilized to decrease abnormal tone, reflexes are less forceful in sitting, gravity will bring knees into flexion (out of lower extremity extensor synergy) and elbows into extension (out of upper extremity decortication). Approximation can be added to normalize tone and promote tonic holding. The patient can be given the feeling of weight shifting by the therapist shifting her own body weight. Trunk elongation can be accomplished by side bending the patient to weight bearing on his elbow on either side, with approximation added to facilitate holding on the weight bearing upper extremity (Figure 5-2).

Patients with strong extensor tone can be rotated and gradually stretched (and

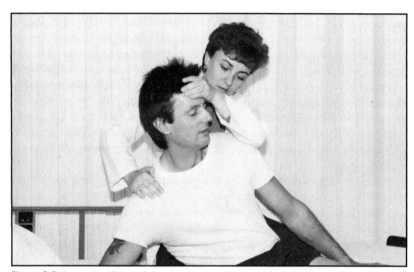

Figure 5-2. Approximation to right upper extremity combined with elongation of the trunk on the left.

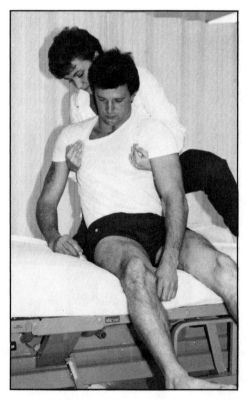

Figure 5-3. Slow rotation with gradual movement into increasing degrees of hip and trunk flexion with the patient demonstrating excessive extensor tone.

maintained) into increased hip and trunk flexion (Figure 5-3). Weight bearing through the lower extremities can be enhanced with approximation through knees. If extensor thrust is a problem, a footstool can be placed under the patient's feet to increase hip flexion (Figure 5-4). Wooden wedges/footboards commonly used in acute care hospitals for hip fracture patients can be used to increase weight bearing and allow positioning of the ankles/knees/hips in increased flexion. A mirror will help the therapist monitor the patient's responses and will provide the patient with visual stimulation for focusing, as well as give visual cueing for feedback to replace or augment losses in the sensory system.

Prone-on-elbows posture can be utilized to promote head and upper trunk stability and to stretch tight hip flexors.

Lower trunk rotation can be used to decrease spasticity, stretch hip adductors, stretch trunk, and provide stimulation and feedback to feet. The therapist can put her hips between the patient's knees for maintained stretch to adductors, place hands on the patient's shoulders to prevent log-rolling, and provide segmental rotation and rhythmic initiation for relaxation of spasticity and

Figure 5-4. Edge-of-bed sitting provides orientation to upright, weight bearing through the spine and lower extremities. The therapist assists with posture and head control.

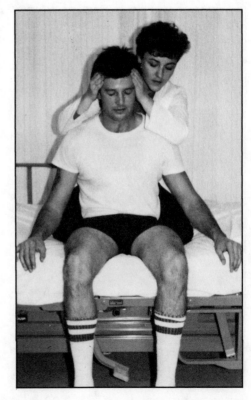

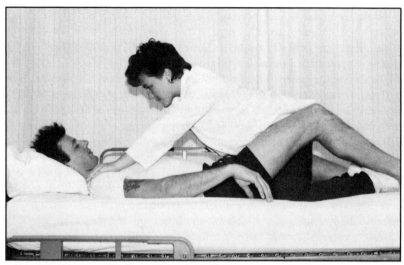

Figure 5-5. The therapist stabilizes the upper trunk with her hands while abducting the patient's lower extremities and rotating the lower trunk with her hips.

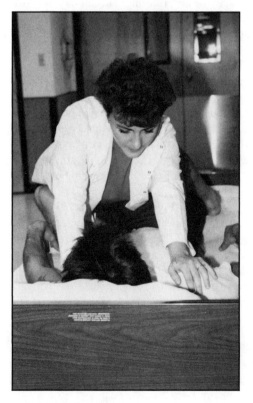

Figure 5-6. Different view of the therapist doing the same as in the previous Figure.

possible increased active movement (Figures 5-5 and 5-6). As the patient relaxes, the lower extremities can be positioned in more or less flexion, depending on the goal. Once relaxed, this is also a good position to facilitate hip abduction and adduction with gravity assisting the abduction.

As soon as the patient is medically able, he should be removed from his room and taken to a variety of settings to increase stimulation. Weight bearing can be accomplished in a standing box, with the use of traditional assistive devices, or with handling of two therapists. Dynamic movement is needed to stimulate righting reactions and can be accomplished by handling of the upper trunk when in static postures on the tilt table, or in the standing box.

Vestibular stimulation is more easily applied in the Physical Therapy Department with the use of rocking boards, rocking chairs, therapy balls, and mechanical lifts. Vestibular stimulation should be applied for brief intervals, allowing time for the system to normalize between stimulation, and the patient should be closely monitored for any adverse effects.

Vestibular stimulation can be applied in conjunction with other treatment techniques. For example, the patient demonstrating decorticate posturing can have air splints applied to both elbows after rhythmical rocking and passive stretching to decrease upper extremity flexor posturing. He can then be positioned prone over a ball and slowly rocked to the head forward position. The prone positioning could encourage lower extremity flexor tone (via symmetrical labyrinthine neck reflex) to decrease extensor posturing. Slow rocking promotes a generalized decrease in tone. The head down position could facilitate flexor tone via the symmetrical tonic neck reflex, and the carotid sinus reflex would encourage a generalized decrease in tone. The therapist can control the patient at the pelvis to counter-rotate in the opposite movement direction of the ball to break up abnormal muscle tone. The movement encourages righting and equilibrium responses as well as head and trunk control. The arc of movement of the ball can be increased to allow brief periods of weight bearing on the extended upper extremities, and then onto the flexed lower extremities, gradually increasing the amount of weight bearing and stretch on the quadriceps to decrease lower extremity extensor spasticity (Figures 5-7, 5-8, and 5-9).

Casting is an important adjunct to therapeutic exercise in preventing the secondary complication of contractures.[1,5,7,11-13] The goals of casting are to prevent deformity, increase range of motion, and inhibit spasticity. Contraindications to casting include unhealed fractures and open wounds. The casting program can be delayed or modified to accommodate the patient's medical condition, need for accessibility of the limb for medical care, and skin condition.

Casting can be carried out in a cast room, the therapy department or at bedside. Equipment needs are listed in Table 5-4. A cylinder cast encompasses only one joint: the elbow in the upper extremities, and the knee in the lower extremities. A long leg cast (LLC) encompasses the knee, ankle, forefoot, and

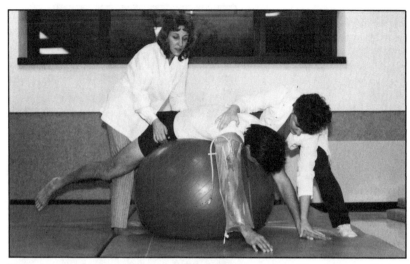

Figure 5-7. Weight bearing on the upper extremities, rotation of the pelvis, carotid sinus reflex, and air splint on right upper extremity will inhibit abnormal muscle tone.

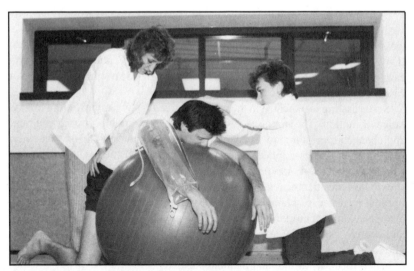

Figure 5-8. Weight bearing through the lower extremities, with approximation added to the hips and with facilitation of head control.

Figure 5-9. Righting reactions can
be facilitated through rocking
while sitting over a bolster.

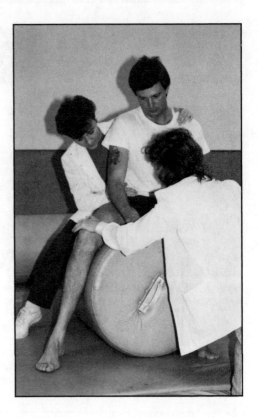

toes. A short-leg cast (SLC) does not encompass the knee. A long arm cast
(LAC) encompasses the elbow, wrist, and fingers (thumb optional). A short arm
cast (SAC) does not include the elbow. Supplies needed specific to each type of
cast are listed in Table 5-5.

Serial casting is indicated in the patient who is already demonstrating limited
range of motion. The initial cast is applied in a comfortable, resting position,
and changed every three to seven days as the spastic muscles adapt to the new
length. Each cast is applied in the "new" resting position without forceful
stretching (Table 5-6, application procedure). Passive range of motion exercises
should be done after the removal of each cast to maintain joint mobility. Once an
optimal position is obtained, indicated by full passive range of motion or no
change in range of motion on subsequent cast removals, the cast can be bivalved
and worn as a splint (Table 5-7, bivalve preparation). A schedule is devised that
allows exercise to the casted extremity while still providing the inhibitory
effects of neutral warmth and maintained stretch.

Therapeutic intervention should now be directed toward facilitation of the
muscles antagonist to the spastic muscles with the ultimate goal of increasing

Table 5-4. Cast Room Equipment Needs.

Treatment table or stretcher
Cast saw, blades, vacuum (optional)
Sink
Working surface
Plastic basin
Cast spreaders
Duckbills
Felt tip markers
Scissors—cast and standard
Padding—Reston®, Temperstick®, Orthopedic felt
Moleskin
Adhesive Tape
Pillows
Two, three, and four inch Stockinet
Three, four, five and six inch roles of padding
Three, four, and five inch rolls of plaster
Rolls of fiberglass tape
Three, four, and five inch plaster splints
Ace® wraps, Velcro® straps, or buckle straps
Weight bearing surfaces—cast shoes, walking heels

Table 5-5. Casting Materials.

Upper Extremities:

SAC	Cylinder Cast	LAC
2 or 3″ stockinet	3″ stockinet	3″ stockinet
Foam/felt padding	Foam/felt padding	Foam/felt padding
2½ rolls 3″ padding	1 roll 3″ padding	2 rolls 3″ padding
3 rolls 3″ plaster	1-2 rolls 4″ padding	1-2 rolls 4″ padding
3″ splints	1 roll 3″ padding	2 rolls 3″ plaster
	2 rolls 4″ plaster	2 rolls 4″ plaster
	4″ splints	3 or 4″ splints

Lower Extremities:

SLC	Cylinder Cast	LLC
3 or 4″ stockinet	4″ stockinet	4″ stockinet
Foam/felt padding	Foam/felt padding	Foam/felt padding
2 rolls 4″ padding	1 roll 4″ padding	2 rolls 4″ padding
1 roll 5″ padding	2 rolls 5″ padding	2 rolls 5″ padding
2 rolls 4″ plaster	1 roll 6″ padding	1 roll 6″ padding
1 roll 5″ plaster	1 roll 4″ plaster	2 rolls 4″ plaster
4″ splints	2 rolls 5″ plaster	2 rolls 5″ plaster
	1 roll 6″ plaster	1 roll 6″ plaster
	5″ splints	4″ splints
		5″ splints

Table 5-6. Cast Application.

1. Assess and document passive range of motion and muscle tone.
2. Apply stockinet without wrinkles, allowing excess to fold back at both ends of cast.
3. Position body part—position must be maintained throughout procedure.
4. Cover all bony prominences with foam or felt padding. Avoid pressure on superficial nerves.
5. Apply rolls of cotton padding in a spiral manner, overlapping one half of the width of the padding. Use narrower widths for distal parts, wider widths for proximal parts.
6. Holding ends, dip plaster in tepid water for approximately 10 seconds (until thoroughly moistened and pasty). Squeeze out excess water without wringing the roll of plaster.
7. Apply plaster in same manner as padding, and smooth throughout procedure. Care should be taken to avoid indenting or pulling the plaster. Keep the borders of the cast consistent in length and thickness.
8. Apply splints as indicated.
9. Fold edges of stockinet over cast borders and secure with final roll of plaster.

Table 5-7. Bivalve Preparation.

1. Cut cast in anterior and posterior sections.
2. Spread halves with cast spreader.
3. Cut padding and remove halves.
4. Strip cast shells.
5. Check for smooth, sharp, or rough ridges.
6. Reapply foam padding to shell.
7. Layer padding consistent with application procedure.
8. Split stockinet and line cast over padding.
9. Tape edges of stockinet around cast edges with moleskin or adhesive.
10. Apply to patient with Ace® wraps, Velcro® straps, or buckle straps.
11. Check fit.
12. Devise schedule.

---

the amount of time out of the cast, and eventually discontinuing the cast.

Serial casting can include the use of drop-out casts. Casts are applied in the resting position and a portion of the cast is cut away to allow range of motion exercises to have gravity assist in increasing range of motion while the cast prevents return to the original position. In the upper extremities, casts may be dropped out at the elbow, wrist, or fingers, depending on the motion desired. To obtain increased elbow extension, the cast can be cut away from the triceps area and around the olecranon process (Figure 5-10).

Gravity can assist elbow extension, while the anterior portion of the cast

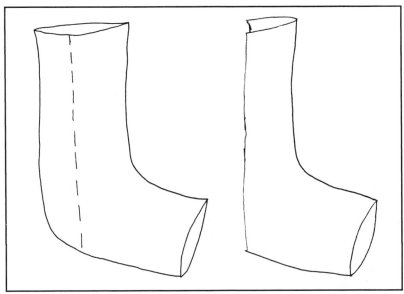

Figure 5-10. Proximal drop-out of UE cylinder casts.

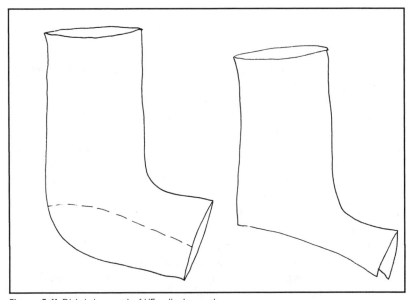

Figure 5-11. Distal drop-out of UE cylinder cast.

prevents flexion. By cutting the cast proximally, the weight of the cast on the forearm will assist gravity in extending the elbow. However, as the elbow extends, the proximal portion of the cast pulls away from the biceps, which is the muscle to be inhibited via neutral warmth, tendon pressure, and maintained stretch. To maintain contact with the biceps muscle, the cast can be cut away distally around the olecranon process and forearm (Figure 5-11).

Gravity can still assist extension of the elbow without the added assistance of the weight of the cast. With the distal cut out, the cast is less likely to slide on the patient, but forearm pronation or supination is more likely. In the proximal drop-out cast, the triceps is accessible for facilitation techniques and modalities.

The wrists and fingers are almost always dropped out to achieve increased extension rather than increased flexion. In the lower extremity, drop-out casts are most frequently used to increase knee flexion or extension, and increase ankle dorsiflexion. Some problems that may occur with drop-out casts include: swelling, increased incidence of skin breakdown secondary to sliding of the cast, or patient movement within the cast. The authors only recommend drop-out casts when family or staff are readily available for frequent range of motion exercises and repositioning.

The Agitated Patient

The agitated patient (Level IV on the Rancho Los Amigos Scale of Cognitive Functioning) is confused, and therefore agitated secondary to disorganization in thought processes leading to exaggerated behavioral responses. The patient is alert but unable to attend to, process, and interpret environmental stimuli. He presents with a variety of responses and behaviors that are a function of his internal confusion.

The primary goal in treatment of the agitated patient is to decrease the intensity, duration, and frequency of agitated responses, and increase attention and response to specific stimuli or tasks.

Treatment of the agitated patient involves reducing environmental stimulation to decrease the patient's confusion and to reinforce appropriate behaviors. The use of medications in this population is controversial, and each patient should be evaluated for appropriate medications on an individual basis.

Some important faotors to keep in mind when dealing with the agitated patient are:

1. The patient cannot be held accountable for his behavior;
2. Confusion causes the patient to be frightened;
3. Increased numbers of people dealing with an agitated patient will usually increase the patient's fear and confusion, and subsequently, increase rather than control his agitation;
4. Restraints usually increase agitation; and

5. The patient is unable to cooperate with therapists, not unwilling.

The patient should be seen in a quiet, nonthreatening environment. Treatment sessions should be brief. The patient should be oriented in a calm, pleasant voice, and all statements should be short and simple. The patient's memory may be severely limited, and he may require frequent, gentle reminders of basic information throughout the treatment sessions and from day to day.

The understanding of the behavioral sequelae of head injury is extremely important to the therapist in the planning of therapeutic activities and assessment of the patient's abilities and disabilities. The therapist's approach to the patient should be based on management of the behavioral problem(s).

In the patient who is confused or disoriented, the therapist will need to reorient the patient as needed, sometimes several times during a session. Patience and provision of information in a calm, nonthreatening manner will help prevent (or at least modify) the acting out or aggressive behavior often seen in the highly confused patient.

Treatment activities should be kept simple and automatic, and the patient should be allowed to succeed at any task.

In treating these patients, physical goals must be secondary to the cognitive goal. The patient's physical abilities will not be functional for the patient if he remains in a state of heightened awareness and confusion. Therefore, any physical therapy treatment that causes discomfort or increased confusion should be deferred until the patient has progressed through this phase of recovery. The patient will usually not tolerate passive weight bearing on a tilt table or in a standing box, as these activities are restrictive to maintain position. The tilt table straps and door on the standing box will probably increase the patient's fear and confusion. Serial casting usually should be deferred as the presence of the cast may increase agitation, and the cast could cause physical harm to the patient and staff.

During treatment, the therapist must present herself in a calm, friendly, and confident manner. Whenever possible, restraints should be removed, but the therapist must be aware of the possibility of physically aggressive behavior from the patient. She should position herself out of reach of the patient or remain in a state of readiness to remove herself from the patient's reach immediately. Have assistance within voice range. A change in behavior can occur without any clear precipitating incident.

It is important for the therapist to assess which environmental factors increase or decrease the patient's agitation. Agitated patients may be calmed by treatment outdoors on a sunny day. The patient may respond to generalized relaxation techniques such as slow stroking down posterior primary rami, slow rocking in a rocking chair, soothing music, and dim lights. In the physically able patient, exercise and walking may calm the patient temporarily. In cases where walking has a soothing affect on the patient, the therapist may need to set aside her goal of adequate weight shifting prior to ambulation.

The patient may participate better in therapy when given physical demonstration of the activity, rather than verbal cues or hands-on assistance. Automatic, overlearned activities will be easier for the patient to succeed at (i.e., throw a ball, walk, ride an exercycle, or roll on a mat).

Many times an agitated period can be redirected by an environmental change (e.g., turn off lights, open window shades, or walk of out room and return). The patient may respond best to topics of interest premorbidly, tapes of familiar voices, and familiar faces.

It is important that all disciplines and family members use a consistent approach with the patient. The patient should be allowed frequent rest periods between activities and throughout the day. All therapeutic intervention should attempt to remove or decrease any stimuli identified as precipitating agitation, and maximize the use of any stimuli that reduce agitation. As the patient develops some basic attention and memory skills, behavior modification programs can be utilized to reinforce appropriate behaviors and redirect inappropriate behaviors.

Midlevel Treatment at Bedside

Many of the procedures outlined at bedside for the low level patient can be carried out with the midlevel patient who presents with limited mobility. Activities can now be geared toward increasing active participation by the patient.

Activities should be structured, repetitive, and easy to accomplish successfully. Rolling activities can now incorporate proprioceptive neuromuscular facilitation diagonals and specific treatment techniques. Bridging can be added to activities at bedside. Depending on patient size and equipment (ventilators, etc.) at bedside, the patient may be able to work in quadruped. Bridging advances the patient out of mass patterns and is a functional activity that can be reinforced by nursing for use of bedpans, and in assisting with bed mobility in preparation for transfers, etc.

The patient can now participate with muscle re-education activities. Directions will have to be short, simple, and noncomplicated. Visual demonstration and feedback visually, tactually, and proprioceptively will be important. Patients at cognitive levels V and VI often present with confusion, and overreact to the stimulus (i.e., react to discomfort as severe pain), have a low frustration tolerance, and may be occasionally verbally and physically abusive.

Modalities can be incorporated into treatment. Biofeedback (EMG) can give the patient added visual and auditory feedback along with the patient's feedback. Electrical stimulation (Functional Electrical Stimulation [FES], Neuromuscular Stimulation [NMS], Variable Muscle Stimulation [VMS]), can be used with patients who do not overreact to stimulation.

CPM units can be applied when the therapist is not present, although this will require frequent monitoring by nursing. Patients cognitively functioning at a Level V or VI are confused, but able to follow commands consistently. They are now able to actively participate with therapeutic interventions that are goal-directed for specific motor abilities as well as cognitive functioning. These patients will present with any or all of the neuromotor complications outlined in Chapter 3.

The Midlevel Patient

Cognitively, the Level V patient is alert, able to follow simple commands with frequent redirection and cueing, and reacts out of proportion on an automatic level. He may confabulate, and lack initiation of functional tasks, but may carry over overlearned activities once started, responds best to self and family, may wander aimlessly, and has continued memory problems.

The primary goals with the confused-inappropriate patient are to decrease confusion, decrease inappropriate behaviors, increase appropriate behaviors, increase orientation, increase attention, improve memory, and improve functional abilities.

The environment should be structured to meet the goals. Initially, limit environmental stimuli to decrease confusion and being distracted. Orientation to person, place, and time should be carried out during each session. All activities should be simply explained and broken down into simple steps. Directions should be one-step commands with added visual and tactile cueing. Activities should allow the patient to succeed. Praise successes and appropriate behaviors. Behavior management plans can be successful at this time when followed consistently.

Physical therapy treatment techniques should be repetitive and in a set sequence to decrease the patient's confusion. Activities need to be explained several times during any given session. Treatment should be provided in the same place, at the same time, and by the same person whenever possible. The patient is now able to participate with therapeutic exercise techniques to promote specific stages of motor control when given simple directions and demonstrations. He will require frequent reminders of the purpose of any casts or adaptive equipment. All staff and family members will need to be informed of the rationale behind such treatments and of the specific cues to consistently give the patient about the need for equipment.

The amount of treatment time requiring the patient's attention should be limited during any one session. As much of the treatment session as possible should focus on facilitating automatic righting and equilibrium responses and on reinforcing normal movement patterns as possible. Activities will need to be switched frequently to maintain the patient's attention.

As the patient progresses, the treatment program can be advanced by increasing the complexity of the activities, decreasing visual, verbal or tactile cues, and increasing distractions.

The patient may now be able to participate with treatment modalities such as EMG biofeedback or electrical stimulation. Given this patient's tendency to overreact to a stimulus, electrical stimulation may be perceived as pain and may not be appropriate until the patient progresses to Level VI.

Biofeedback training should be initiated on the least affected extremity to provide the patient with the easiest, most successful method of learning. Carryover will be minimal, so directions must be simple, repetitive, and consistent from day to day.

Functional activities should be taught in components. The therapist can carry out the activity with the patient completing only one component initially, and as each step is mastered, gradually placing increasing demands on the patient (one step at a time). As these patients have a limited capacity for new learning, and limited carryover, they should not be instructed to use devices that will not be necessary later on (i.e., do not teach ambulation with a walker and then with a cane).

The Level VI patient is still confused but appropriate. He is able to follow simple commands consistently, is inconsistently oriented, is demonstrating improvements in memory, can attend to activities with structure, responds appropriately to discomfort and in proportion to the stimulus, and shows carryover for previously learned tasks. The patient's behaviors are now goal-directed.

The goals of treatment are to increase orientation, increase selective attention, increase initiation, improve planning and sequencing abilities, and increase functional abilities.

The patient is now able to participate with all physical therapy interventions and may be challenged by reducing structure through increasing complexity of commands, increasing number of steps in a procedure, and varying the sequence of activities. The patient may be able to learn all steps of an activity with repetition. A written, step-by-step sequence can be provided for the patient for a functional activity. The patient can review the list, and then perform the activity. The patient may now be able to self-cue and self-monitor for some steps of the activity requiring less cueing from the therapist. Functional activities will need to be practiced in a variety of settings as there will not be carryover from one situation to another.

Therapeutic exercise programs can be more varied and place increasing physical and cognitive demands on the patient. Emphasis can be placed on more subtle techniques to improve the quality of movement.

High-Level Patients

The high-level patient who presents with moderate to severe physical impairments will need to be involved with treatment activities as outlined for low and mid-level patients. The Level VII patient (automatic-appropriate) can be frustrating for the therapist because he lacks insight into his deficits and therefore may need maximal encouragement to participate with his rehabilitation.

The Level VIII patient is purposeful and appropriate and can be treated like all neurological patients from a physical standpoint.

Given the subtlety of cognitive deficits in patients of these levels, they should be referred as soon as possible for appropriate rehabilitation. Activities now will be geared toward functional prevocational, vocational, and community re-entry.

The Family

As the head injured patient is suddenly and unexpectedly thrown into a dramatic life change, so too is the family. They are faced with the need to make many decisions, which even a person in a noncrisis situation would have much difficulty making.

When looking at statistics, they show the average victim of head injury to be a young male between the ages of 15 and 35.[14] The devastation to the family unit is apparent. The family is often faced with the permanent disability of a child who the day before had their entire life ahead of them, or a young husband and father who may no longer be able to fill the role of husband or father.

It is important for the therapist to remember that the family is also a victim of a head injury, and that they will need much education and guidance to become survivors.

The stress experienced by the family members in their attempt to remain supportive to the patient is immense. This stress, however, is usually not short-lived. Oddy and associates[15] found that families may maintain these high stress levels up to a year or longer after the family member's injury.

The family of a head injured patient is a family in crisis. They are often unable to cope with the patient's needs and personality changes so often associated with brain injury. It is at this point that one sees the family beginning to reorganize around the patient's needs, conditions, and moods. In doing so, they are becoming a dysfunctional system as the members are giving up their normal roles to focus solely on the injured member. This places additional stress on all family members.

If the family system falls apart, it can have a tremendous effect on the patient's progress. The outcome of rehabilitation is highly dependent not only on the patient's abilities, but also on family resources: emotional, physical, and financial.

Families dealing with a severely injured member often go through a grieving process similar to that which a family goes through when a member dies.[16] Unlike the family whose member dies, the family of a head injured patient may go through this process several times. The other major difference is the need of the family in the case of the head injured patient to adjust instead of accept.[17]

In the early stages of recovery, denial is usually the primary defense mechanism used by the family.[18] It is important for the therapist working with the patient in the early stages of care, including early rehabilitation, that for the family, denial is hope.[18] It is a normal reaction which allows them to cope with an overwhelming situation.

While the therapist is not often involved immediately in the crisis which surrounds the onset of injury, her early involvement with the patient gives her an excellent opportunity to offer ongoing support and education, and the opportunity to allow for ventilation and constructive activities.

When aiding the family to work through their denial, it is important to allow them time to process new information. They are being barraged with medical and technical information which is totally foreign to them. They will need constant and understanding repetition. Often, writing down explanations will help their understanding. It is important to realize that they may ask the same questions over and over. Answer these questions honestly without taking away their need for hopefulness.

The therapist can provide a vehicle for emphathic listening. The family needs to verbalize their fears and hopes. This provides them with a sort of "reality testing."

As stated earlier in this section, denial is often followed by grief. This is a process which cannot be rushed if it is to be appropriately resolved. As therapists, we must allow the family the freedom to resolve their grief in spite of our often "let's get the show on the road" attitude.

To help the family work through this process, we can point out any gains which the patient may be making and explain the significance of these gains in the recovery process, while at the same time not inflating their significance.

Grief often alternates with the next step in the adjustment process, which is depression. In the family of the head injured patient, depression often manifests itself as loss of hope and hopelessness. If the family is not able to resolve these feelings, it can lead to fundamental unhealthy changes in the family structure.

Anger often replaces depression. This is probably the most difficult, but most important factor, for the therapist to help the family deal with. Oftentimes, we forget that the anger being displayed by the family is not directed at us personally, but at the situation over which they (the family) has no control.

In dealing with the family who is angry, the therapist must remember that it is fear which makes the family angry: fear their family member may not live, may not recover, and will never be the same. The therapist must help the family confront their fears, and allow them to verbalize their anger. Again, highlight gains the patient is making. Make realistic short-term goals for the patient and family.

Getting the family involved with the patient's therapy can prove extremely valuable for both the family and the patient. The family should be encouraged to participate as members of the therapy team. They can be taught therapeutic techniques for use with their patient. Oftentimes, because of the familiarity with the family, the patient may respond better to a family member. Encourage them to make audiotapes for the times they cannot be there. Make the family feel that their efforts are a viable part of the therapy process.

Education of the family is a primary role of the therapist in both the acute and rehabilitation settings. The family needs to be provided with ongoing relevant and accurate information. This will help the family to develop realistic expectations. The provision of this information also puts the therapist in a position to offer anticipatory guidance which may help the family to resolve their grief process in a more healthy manner.

In the end, the therapist plays an important role in helping the family adapt and adjust to their new roles by providing the continuing education, support, time, and attention to identify, practice, and integrate these roles which will allow them to become survivors instead of victims.

References

1. Boughton A, Ciesla N: Physical therapy management of the head injured patient in the intensive care unit. Top Acute Care Trauma Rehabil 1986;1:1-18.
2. Cope ND, Hall K: Head injury rehabilitation: Benefit of early intervention. Arch Phys Med Rehabil 1982;63:433.
3. Jeannett B, Teasdale G: Management of Head Injury. FA Davis Co, Philadelphia, 1981.
4. Jeannett B: Scale and scope of the problem. In Rosenthal M, Griffith ER, Bond, MR, et al (Eds): Rehabilitation of the Head Injured Adult. FA Davis Co, Philadelphia, 1983.
5. Carr JH, Shepher RB: Physiotherapy in Disorders of the Brain. William Heinemann Medical Books Ltd, London, 1980.
6. Nelson AJ: Strategies for improving motor control. In Rosenthal M, Griffith ER, Bond MR, et al (Eds): Rehabilitation of the Head Injured Adult. FA Davis Co, Philadelphia, 1983.
7. Perrin JC: Head injury. In Molnar GE (Ed): Pediatric Rehabilitation. Williams & Wilkins Co, Baltimore, 1985.
8. Davis CW, Kerrick RC: Treatment of head injured patients in the acute stages. Clinical Management 1985;5:16-23.
9. Booth BJ, Doyle M, Montgomery J: Serial casting for the management of spasticity in the head injured adult. Phys Ther 1983;63:18-24.
10. Griffith ER: Spasticity. In Rosenthal M, Griffith ER, Bond MR, et al (Eds): Rehabilitation of the Head Injured Adult. FA Davis Co, Philadelphia, 1983.

11. Shaw R: Persistent vegetative state: Principles and techniques for seating and positioning. Head Trauma Rehabil 1986;1:31-37.
12. Sullivan PE, Markos PD, Minor MA: An Integrated Approach to Therapeutic Exercise theory and Clinical Application. Reston Publishing Co Inc, Reston, Va, 1982.
13. Harris FA: Facilitation techniques and technological adjuncts in therapeutic exercise. In Basmajian JV (Ed): Therapeutic Exercise. Ed 4. Williams & Wilkins Co, Baltimore, 1984.
14. Anderson DW, McLaurin RL (Eds): Report on National Head and Spinal Cord Injury Survey, conducted for the National Institute of Neurological and Communicative Disorders and Stroke. J Neurosurg 1980;S-1(suppl)(November).
15. Oddy M, Humphrey M, Uteley D: Stresses upon the relatives of head injured patients. Br J Psychol 1978;133:507.
16. Pawer PW, Dell Orto AE: Role of the Family in the Rehabilitation of the Physically Disabled. University of Maryland Press. Baltimore, 1980.
17. Kubler-Ross E: On Death and Dying. Macmillan Press, New York, 1969.
18. Epperson M: Families in sudden crisis: Process and intervention in a critical care center. Soc Work Health Care 1977;2:265.

Chapter 6

ASSESSMENT FOR LONG-TERM REHABILITATION POTENTIAL

At some point during the acute hospital stay, a determination will need to be made regarding the possibility of post-hospital rehabilitation. This may occur at any stage of the patient's recovery process. In a small community hospital, this may be as soon as medical stability is achieved; in a larger medical center, it may be after a trial of acute short-term rehabilitation.

The basic goal of ongoing rehabilitation is to attempt to give to the head injured patient the highest quality of life possible. While attempts can be made to assess probable outcome, it remains questionable at best. Given the inability to give a definite prognosis, the authors feel that whenever possible, the patient needs to be given an opportunity for rehabilitation, especially if the patient is less than one year post onset. In assessing a head injured patient for continued rehabilitation, there are several important factors to keep in mind. These include:

1. Assessment of severity of injury on admission;
2. Assessment of residual physical, cognitive, and emotional deficits remaining during recovery;
3. Assessment of rehabilitative attempts during initial hospitalization; and
4. Assessment of the effects of the injury on the family unit.

The Low Level Patient

When specifically evaluating the low level patient for long-term rehabilitation, several factors need to be considered. These include medical instability, level of awareness, physical impairment, extent of injury, age, time post onset, therapeutic intervention to date, present functional level, potential for rehabilitation, and expected outcome. Improvement in neurological status, as seen by changes in the Glasgow Coma Soale (as previously discussed), provide a good early basis for predicting outcome and assessing the potential for rehabilitation. As the patient's Glasgow Coma Scale score improves, it is reflective of the patient's ability to react with and respond to the environment, albeit in a limited manner.

Medical Stability

A patient's medical stability will affect the extent of participation in a full rehabilitation program. Many times patients are transferred to rehabilitation facilities while experiencing continuing medical difficulties, including unstable cardiovascular system irregularities, thermal regulation difficulties, poorly controlled seizure activity, intermittent respiratory complications/infections, and severe negative nitrogen balance due to poor nutrition.

While the above problems would not totally preclude transfer to a rehabilitation setting, it would decrease the intensity of the program in which the patient was able to participate. While most rehabilitation facilities are not staffed or equipped to handle medically unstable patients, rehabilitation units in acute care facilities would be an appropriate placement option for such patients.

There is a current trend for freestanding rehabilitation facilities to establish "special care" units for the care of patients with some medical problems in which a more intensive level of medical care is provided in conjunction with appropriate therapy programs.

A careful review of attempted therapeutic intervention to achieve medical stability and increased endurance should be made. If a progressive program as outlined in Chapter 5 has been followed without progress, then the likelihood of improvement in an intensive rehabilitation program is guarded. However, if little or no attempt at therapeutic intervention has been made, then the patient should be placed in an intensive therapy program.

Limiting the patient's therapy interaction to that which occurs at bedside when he presents with continuing fevers, pneumonias, decubiti, orthostatic hypotension, and contracture may well be perpetuating those complications through lack of aggressive management.

Two highly significant factors in determining the low level patient's appropriateness for intensive rehabilitation are age and time post onset. It has been consistently reported that the younger the patient, the better the outcome.[1] Statistics have shown the best outcomes in patients with essentially similar injuries in the under 20 age group. There is a corresponding final decrease in outcome with each decade of increased age.

When considering time post onset, one must again look at type of and response to therapeutic intervention in the acute care setting. The patient who remains in an unresponsive state for three months is unlikely to achieve a good recovery.[2] Maximal spontaneous recovery occurs within the first six months, with continued, slower recovery occurring during the next year. Still slower, more subtle recovery can occur over several years.[3] According to Cope and Hall,[4] animal studies have shown that final functional outcome and rate of recovery with central nervous system insults are directly related to early and continuous intervention as well as to a stimulating environment. Human studies have shown similar results. However, unlike in the animal studies, researcher have been unable to control all the factors. Although the low level patient who is less than six months post onset is highly appropriate for a rehabilitation program, it should be noted here that the time frame of six months should be used only as a guideline. Factors such as medical instability or a deprived environment must be taken into consideration. For example, the patient that is 6½ months post onset, who had numerous medical complications and had received little or no therapeutic intervention would also be an appropriate candidate for a trial of intensive rehabilitation.

Severity of Injury

Several parameters are used when assessing severity of injury. The three primary factors are length of coma, site, and type of injury. Length of coma can be correlated with site and type of injury.

Length of Coma

There are various definitions of coma. The main theme of all definitions of the state of coma is the patient's total noninteraction with the environment, such as is seen in patients who lack a sleep/wake cycle on EEG testing (Chapter 4).

While literature indicates that a sleeplike coma usually lasts a maximum of four weeks, the patient in a vegetative state may show only minimal interaction (i.e., arousal) with the environment. The longer the vegetative state persists, the less likely it is that the patient will progress within a rehabilitation program (according to Jeannett and Teasdale).[5] The shorter the duration of "true coma," the better the probability of making significant gains.[5]

When evaluating the low level patient for rehabilitation, it is imperative to recognize that rehabilitation, in general, is a learning process and the patient (even low level) must be able to interact with his environment. However, low level patients who are eventually expected to be discharged to home, should usually receive intensive rehabilitation to prepare the patient for home care and to educate the caregivers.

Site of Injury

Site of injury has a significant impact on prognosis and ability to participate in a rehabilitation program. Specific areas of the brain affect different functional areas from arousal to insight and judgment, as shown in Chapter 2. For evaluation of the low level patient, site of injury should be viewed from how diffuse the injury is. This can be assessed by a careful review of diagnostic studies. Bi-hemispheric damage, enlarged ventricles, midline shift of the ventricles, and space-occupying lesions can be documented on initial and subsequent CT scans.[6] If the patient has been in the acute care unit for several months, the scans may also show the presence or absence of cortical atrophy. All the aforementioned factors would tend toward a guarded rehabilitation prognosis. In descending order, a worse prognosis is associated with subdural hematoma, diffuse injury without focal lesion, and epidural hematoma. A midline shift of greater than 4 mm is associated with a poor outcome.[7]

Cerebral injury has had a better prognosis than brainstem injury in some of the literature.[7]

Another diagnostic study to assist in determining the severity of injury are evoked potential studies. Case studies presented by Rappaport[8] show that evoked potential patterns can not only provide information on the patient's condition, but also on ultimate outcome and appropriateness for an intensive rehabilitation program. Patients whose visual and somatosensory evoked potential studies were moderately or markedly abnormal may be expected to show reasonable progress.

Type of Injury

When using type of injury in assessing a patient's potential for rehabilitation, it is important to keep in mind the amount of damage caused by the various injuries.

A patient who has sustained brain injury due to hypoxia (i.e., cardiac/respiratory arrest) will have a more extensive, diffuse axonal injury, which causes decreased plasticity. The patient with a severe closed head injury caused by deceleration (i.e., motor vehicle) may also show widespread damage as a result of the brain's continued movement when the skull is decelerated. Unlike the anoxic injury, however, there does not appear to be as severe damage to the brain's plasticity. This is probably related to continuing oxygenation of the brain.

In a patient who has sustained a local injury (i.e., blow to the head), most of the cerebral damage will be localized below the point of impact. In an open or penetrating injury such as a bullet wound, the amount of damage will be dependent on the missile or fragment tract.

(Refer to Appendix L for an evaluation form for post acute rehabilitation of the low level patient.)

The Agitated Patient

When assessing the agitated patient for post-acute rehabilitation, there are several points which need to be considered. Most important are the length of coma, degree of hyperactivity, and disorganization.

Length of Coma

It is generally accepted that the duration of agitation is in direct proportion to the duration of coma. While not all patients who have sustained head injuries go through periods of agitation, length of coma may be useful in determining how long a patient can be expected to exhibit agitated behaviors. If the patient has been in a prolonged state of agitation, prognosis for significant improvement in a rehabilitation facility would be highly guarded.

Hyperactivity and Disorganization

The degree of hyperactivity and disorganization can be assessed by examining the number of outbursts in a given period, duration of the outbursts, and any factors which may have precipitated or defused it. The patient demonstrating intermittent periods of agitation may show some ability to participate in a therapy program during periods of decreased agitation.[9] Some agitated patients may have only brief outbursts and when given a "time out" (i.e., reduction of stimulation) may return to a more appropriate behavior pattern.

Environmental factors have a profound effect on the brain injured patient's ability to process input. The agitated patient who is surrounded by unfamiliar equipment, faces, sounds, and procedures is more likely to respond with confusion and aggression. It is imperative to note the patient's responses within a quiet, controlled environment in which stimulation has been minimized or eliminated. Close attention should be paid to the effects of withdrawal of each stimulant.

Cognition

If the agitated patient is demonstrating some periods of confused, nonagitated behavior, it is important to assess his level of basic cognitive abilities. Assessment should be directed toward attention span, memory functioning, and language abilities. Even during periods of outbursts, some cognitive abilities may be apparent. The content of verbal expression may give an indication of intact language functioning and underlying cognitive abilities which may have been masked by the patient's state of internal confusion. Between periods of aggressive and disinhibited behavior, evaluation of basic memory can indicate the beginning of moving out of PTA. The presence of PTA (the absence of day-to-day memory of events or people) increases the agitation, and return of memory functioning would indicate the potential to control "disinhibition" and modify behaviors.

Severe depression of cognitive functioning in these patients necessitates a close review of any psychotropic medications. Medications prescribed to control agitation usually must be administered in excessively high doses to obtain the desired effect.[10,11]

Management

Assessment of management techniques utilized during the hospitalization period will allow the reviewer to look at possible avenues of intervention in the rehabilitation setting.

Environmental controls, as discussed in Chapters 4 and 5, are essential to promoting recovery through the agitated stage. If the environment has been overstimulating, then the patient may benefit from a highly structured rehabilitation program utilizing environmental modification and behavior management techniques. Conversely, if these techniques have already been attempted in a consistent manner, it is unlikely that continued rehabilitation will result in significant benefit.

The use of restraints, both physical and chemical, must also be noted. Rao, et al[4] have reported some positive results with psychotropic medications, although their usage may add to the patient's internal confusion and disorientation,[3] along with clouding of the sensorium. However, the use of physical restraints consistently adds to the patient's confusion and subsequently may prolong agitation. These patients may be appropriate for continued rehabilitation by titration of medication, and provision of a safe environment with a consistent approach in order to build on the patient's emerging cognitive and perceptual abilities.

The assessment tool for evaluating the agitated patient has been geared to the most frequently seen medical, functional, cognitive, and behavioral problems seen in these patients, along with variables such as therapy involvement, use of restraints, number and duration of outbursts. This should give a thorough overview of the patient's level of agitation and when viewed from all areas, provide a basis for determining rehabilitation potential (Appendix M).

Assessing the Midlevel Patient

In assessing the midlevel patient for continued post-hospitalization rehabilitation, it is important to remember the behaviors consistent with these cognitive levels. The Level V patient is confused and inappropriate, the Level VI patient is confused and appropriate. Both patients will require a structured environment and consistent approaches to decrease confusion, gradually decrease structure, and increase independence. Almost categorically, these patients require an intensive interdisciplinary inpatient rehabilitation program specifically designed for head injury rehabilitation. Therefore, assessment of the midlevel patient is directed not at whether rehabilitation is indicated, but which type of facility is most appropriate for the patient.

Assessing the High Level Patient

Patients who are demonstrating behaviors consistent with Levels VII and VIII are appropriate and automatic or purposeful. These patients are independent for daily routines, and therefore may mistakenly be discharged home without bringing the patients to their fullest potential. These patients cannot return to work and society without continued intervention. Again, as with the midlevel patients, assessment is aimed at choosing the most appropriate rehabilitation program. These patients may be able to live at home and go to outpatient programs for cognitive or physical rehabilitation. The cognitive deficits in these patients may be very subtle, and it is extremely important that their follow-up be provided by professionals and programs equipped to deal with these problems. These patients may require specialized evaluations to determine rehabilitation needs and to plan programs that will assist each patient to returning as a functional member of society. This specialized type of evaluation can outline a stepwise program of initial rehabilitation needs, vocational training or education, and transitional and ultimate living setting.

As with all head injured patients, the mid and high level patients should be evaluated with regard to severity of injury, residual deficits, recovery curves, progress to date, rehabilitative efforts in the acute care setting, and assessment of the patient's support system (Appendix N).

Assessment will give the therapist a good idea as to the appropriateness of initiating or continuing rehabilitation.

When initiating discharge planning, one must have a clear picture of the variety of services available, their location, and admission requirements, as well as the patient's abilities, limitations, and prognosis.

The high level patient who has made a rapid recovery from a mild head injury may be able to bypass continued inpatient physical and cognitive treatment and be referred directly to an outpatient program specializing in vocational rehabilitation. For those higher level patients requiring continued physical and cognitive rehabilitation, a decision should be made as to whether an inpatient, outpatient, or in-home program is most appropriate.

The patient who has minimal physical deficits, but continues to have difficulties in the areas of cognition would need a program which would focus on remediation of cognitive factors interfering with functional abilities and independence. Coversely, in the patient who continues to exhibit moderate to severe physical limitations, assessment for continued rehabilitation would focus on the patient's abilities to learn alternate methods of mobility and environmental control.

An assessment of the patient whose level of cognition and physical functioning remains severely impaired would focus on placement in a facility which could provide the needed medical management and intensive cognitive stimulation, as well as continued physical rehabilitation.

Assessment of appropriate plaoement for the agitated patient would be geared toward a program which would provide the needed high levels of structure (possibly one-on-one coverage), behavior management programs, and continued cognitive and physical rehabilitation. Other factors affecting assessment of an appropriate placement would include family issues, location, and availability of appropriate facilities. Available funding sources of payment and the patient's willingness to participate in a continued therapy program also come into play.

Placement Options

When working with the head injured patient, appropriate post-hospital treatment is an extremely important issue. The placement selected must be able to meet the ongoing needs of the individual patient. Like the treatment plan, placement must be individualized to the needs of the patient. Usual placement options would include inpatient rehabilitation, outpatient treatment, or day treatment programs, home based rehabilitation, vocational program placement, and long-term placement.

Each of these placement possibilities provides different services and treatment regimes. The problem is choosing which placement is most appropriate for the patient. The therapist can and should play an important role in helping to establish which option is most appropriate.

Inpatient Treatment

Inpatient treatment facilities are probably the most familiar to the therapist. They provide ongoing rehabilitation to the patient in a setting often similar to that of the hospital. When looking into inpatient rehabilitation placement, it is important to closely review the services available, staff qualifications, and if a program is available to meet the specific rehabilitation needs of the head injured patient.

It is important to remember that as the therapist who may have had the most contact with the patient, the family will often turn to you, along with the social worker, in discharge planning to help them determine the appropriateness of their placement choices.

The following is a list of questions which you could advise the family to ask when continued inpatient rehabilitation is the treatment of choice. While they are not the only questions that could be asked, they would help the family in formulating an informed decision.

1. What level patient does the facility accept? (Many facilities accept only patients of a Level V or higher).
2. Do they treat only head injured patients? If not, how many head injured patients do they usually treat at a given time?
3. Does the facility offer a full range of physical, occupational, speech, recreational, and psychologioal therapy services?
4. Is the facility accredited by an agency such as the Commission on Accreditation of Rehabilitation Facilities (CARF)?
5. Does the facility provide specialized programs to meet the needs of the head injured patient? These would include intensive stimulation programs for the low level patient, behavior management programs for the agitated patient, etc.
6. Is the facility able to provide community orientation programs for the higher level patient so that he may begin to learn to reintegrate himself into society?
7. Does the facility allow the family to fully participate in the patient's therapy program and do they, in fact, encourage it?
8. Does the facility have the appropriate equipment and adequate staff to provide the services they state are available?
9. Is the program overseen by a physiatrist, neurologist, or neuro-psychologist?
10. Should medical emergencies arise, are they able to be handled adequately?
11. Do the patients and families already at this facility seem pleased?

The final, and possibly most important question the therapist should encourage the family to ask is one which they (the family) must ask themselves: are they comfortable with the facility and will they be comfortable leaving their family member in the care of the staff? Unless the family is comfortable with the decision, neither they nor the patient will make gains toward recovery and adjustment.

This is often the most difficult question for the family. Oftentimes they are required to select a program which is located hundreds of miles from their home in order that their family member is involved in the most appropriate program.

Outpatient and Day Treatment Programs

Another possibility for post-hospital treatment is outpatient or day treatment programs. These programs provide services to those patients for whom intensive inpatient rehabilitation is either not appropriate or unavailable for whatever reasons.

The patient most likely to be involved in an outpatient program is one who is able to function either independently or with minimal assistance in the community, but continues to need remediation activities for remaining physical or cognitive deficits. An individualized program is devised, often based on the recommendations of the therapist in the acute care setting. Therapy is usually limited to two or three sessions daily or several times per week. The family will need to provide stucure and reinforcement at home whenever the patient is not at a therapy session.

Unfortunately, this is often the only option available, even to the patient who requires more intensive rehabilitation due to insurance or other funding limitations. When this is the case, as full a therapy schedule as possible should be devised by the therapist and sent to the outpatient clinic.

Day treatment programs are a relatively new development in post-acute treatment of the head injured patient. While similar to outpatient therapy in that the patient does not stay in the facility to receive therapy, they offer a much more intensive level of treatment, frequently offering as much as five to six hours of therapy daily. This allows the patient needing extensive continuing therapy to live in the less confining situation of his home while receiving the required therapy. This is an ideal situation for the family who wishes to care for the patient at home. It allows the family to achieve some sense of normalcy in that family members can continue to carry on regular daytime activities such as work or school, and to provide for the patient's needs in the evening.

While to date there are not many day treatment programs, their popularity as viable placement options should grow based on their ability to meet the needs of the patient and family in a cost-effective manner.

Home Treatment

More frequently, home based care is being selected for post-acute care. This could be due to either family wishes or to necessity due to lack of funding for other types of rehabilitative care. Recent trends[1] are showing more families opting for home care than in the past, regardless of the level of care required by the patient. In fact, the number of families opting to take the low level patient home appears to be increasing.[1] Often, the family believes, and rightly so, that they can provide the best environment, especially when faced with the possibility of placing a child or young adult in a long-term placement facility.

If this is the option chosen by the family, the physical therapist's role will be of prime importance. It will be up to the therapist not only to devise an appropriate program of home therapy, but also to teach family members how to provide such treatments. This can be a long process, requiring much understanding and patience on the part of the physical therapist.

In addition to the home treatment plan, the physical therapist should assist the family in determining what types of equipment may be needed. The therapist may want to recommend such equipment as exercise mats, a tilt table, or standing box. The physical therapist may also work with the occupational therapist in devising any needed home modifications and environmental control systems. A teaching record should be devised, so that an accurate record of teaching may be kept (Table 6-1).

After discharge, follow-up contact by the therapist can be of tremendous help to the family to provide assurance and reinforcement.

Long-term Placement

In the authors' opinion, long-term placement or placement in a nursing home should always be the last possible option when seeking placement. Few nursing homes (although there are some) are equipped or staffed to handle the problems of the head injured patient. Many nursing homes will not even consider admitting a young head injured patient.

Should nursing home placement be the only option or the choice of the family, they will need much support. Here again, the therapist can devise a treatment plan that can be taught to the family for use in the long-term care facility. Often just knowing that they can continue a range of motion or basic ADL program will help the family cope.

As with the home treatment program, follow-up calls to the family and facility to offer support and guidance can prove to be invaluable.

Vocational Programs

For the high level patient who will require only a minimal therapy program on discharge, referral to a vocational program may be appropriate. If a prevocational (or vocational) assessment has been completed during the patient's acute hospital stay, the therapist may have already been working on tasks which would allow the patient to return to his prior occupation. If residual motor deficits such as poor balance or impaired short-term memory and attention span deficits are present, return to previous employment may be impossible.

In this case, referral to the local Office or Bureau of Vocational Rehabilitation would be indicated. Often these agencies are able to place the head injured patient in an appropriate vocational re-educational program to prepare him for employment in a new area. Many of these programs are funded through county and state agencies and provide the patient with the opportunity to again become a functional member of society and regain his position in the family hierarchy.

Funding

In the preceding sections on placement, funding or the lack of the same was frequently mentioned. While we all want our patients to participate in the most

Table 6-1. Family Teaching Record.

Date	Task/Objective	Family Observation	Family Assist With Task	Family Demonstration	Therapist Comment	Therapist/Family Init.
9/7	Stand/pivot trans.	X			Mother uncomfortable w/ attempting S/P transfer at this time.	SM/PT DB
9/9	As above	X	X		Mom assisted w/ transfer. Reminded about proper body position.	SM/PT DB
9/10	As above			X	Mom performed S/P transfer. Did well. Will have her do transfers on unit w/superv. for 3 days to become more comfortable w/procedure.	SM/PT DB
9/12	Proper w/c position w/adaptive equipment.	X	X		Reinforced imp. of proper position and body alignment.	SM/PT DB

appropriate post-acute rehabilitation program possible, this is often not possible. The problem of funding for continued rehabilitation is one we are becoming acutely aware of.

Funding for rehabilitation is usually provided for by a third party payor, such as a health insurance or automobile liability insurance carrier. Oftentimes, especially in health insurance policies, coverage for rehabilitation is extremely limited or not available.

Some policies which do allow for post-hospital rehabilitation may have dollar limitations on them. Much of this can be used during the patient's acute hospital stay, especially if there have been many medical complications. This dollar limit applies not only to health insurance policies, but many automobile insurances also. For example, motorists in the state of New York may purchase no-fault automobile insurance for $25,000, $50,000, or $100,000. Once these monies are exhausted, unless there is a health insurance policy for back up, no further funds are available. Several states, however, do have unlimited auto no-fault policies. These policies cover the appropriate and necessary needs of the patient for as long as necessary.

Another type of insurance which funds for post-hospital rehabilitation is worker's compensation. Whether or not there is a cap on these funds is dependent on the individual state in which the policy is written. These funds are often closely watched over by rehabilitation specialists who determine whether or not continued rehabilitation is warranted. These specialists are usually rehabilitation nurses and counselors who work closely with the therapist in determining an appropriate plan of care.

Medical assistance is another possible source of funding. For the patient with no other insurance, or for the patient who has exhausted all other insurance coverage, medical assistance may pay for post-hospital rehabilitation. The main problem with medical assistance is that because of its often low rates of reimbursement, it is often prohibitive for a rehabilitation facility to have a large number of these patients at any given time.

While the therapist is not normally active in placement and funding issues, it is important to be aware of these in order to assist the family in their decision-making process and to support them once a decision is made regarding placement.

References

1. Brink JD, Imbus C, Woo-Sam J: Physical recovery after severe closed head trauma in children and adolescents. J Pediatr 1980;97:721.
2. Bartkowski HM, Lovely MP: Prognosis in coma and the persistent vegetative state. Head Trauma Rehabil 1986;1(1):1-5.
3. Kigashi K, Halano M, Aluko S, et al: Five year follow up study of patients with persistent vegetative state. J Neurol Neurosurg Psychiatry 1981;44:552.

4. Cope DN, Hallo K: Head injury rehabilitation: Benefit of early intervention. Arch Phys Med Rehabil 1982;63:433.
5. Jeannett B, Teasdale G: Assessment of coma and impaired consciousness. Lancet 1984;2:81.
6. Perini S, Beltramello A, Pusat ML, et al: Central nervous system trauma: Head Injuries. In Buonanno FS: Neurologic Clinics. Vol 2, No 4. WB Saunders Co, Philadelphia, 1984.
7. Rao N, Jellinek H, Harvey R, et al: CT head scans as predictors of rehabilitation outcome. Arch Phys Med Rehabil 1984;65:1980.
8. Rappaport M: Brain evoked potentials in coma and the vegetative state. Head Trauma Rehabil 1986;1(1):15.
9. Klauber KW, Ward-McKinley C: Managing behavior in the patient with traumatic brain injury. Top Acute Care Trauma Rehabil 1986;1(1):48.
10. Bobath BS, Doyle M, Malkmus D: Meeting the challenge of the agitated patient. In Rehabilitation of the Head Injured Adult: Comprehensive Management. Professional Staff Association, Rancho Los Amigos Hospital, Downey, Calif, 1979.
11. Rao N, Jellinek HM, Woolston DC: Agitation in closed head injury: Haloperidol effects on rehabilitation outcome. Arch Phys Med Rehabil 1985;66:30.

BIBLIOGRAPHY

Alexandre A: Cognitive outcome and early indices of severity of head injury. J Neurosurg 1983;59:751-761.

American Physical Therapy Association: Electromyographic Biofeedback: An Anthology. Alexandria, Va, 1983.

Annepers JF, et al: The incidence, causes and secular trends of head trauma in Olmstead County, Minnesota, 1935-1974. Neurology 1980;30:912-919.

Annepers JF, et al: Seizures after head trauma: A population study. Neurology 1980;30:683-689.

Basmajian JV (Ed): Therapeutic Exercise. Ed 4. Williams & Wilkins Co, Baltimore, 1984.

Bates B: A Guide to Physical Examination. JB Lippincott Co, Philadelphia, 1974.

Becker DP, et al: The outcome from severe head injury with early diagnosis and intensive management. J Neurosurg 1977;47:491.

Ben Yishay Y, Diller L: Rehabilitation of cognitive and perceptual defects in people with traumatic brain damage. J Rehabil Res Dev 1981;4(2):208-210.

Ben Yishay Y, Rattok J, Ross B, et al: Rehabilitation of cognitive and perceptual deficits in people with traumatic brain damage: A five year clinical research study. In Working Approaches to Remediation of Cognitive Deficits in Brain Damaged Persons, (Rehabilitation Monograph No. 64). New York University Medical Center: Institute of Rehabilitation Medicine, 1982, pp 127-176.

Ben-Yishay Y, Rattok J, Ross B: Rehabilitation in cognitive and perceptual deficits in people with traumatic brain damage: A five year clinical research study. In: Working Approach to Remediation of Cognitive Deficits in Brain Damage. (Rehabiltation Monograph No. 64). New York University Medical Center: Institute of Rehabiltation Medicine, 1982, pp 127-176.

Berkovsky D: Psychological effects of closed head injury. Neurosurgical Nursing 1972;IV(2).

Bolin R: Sensory deprivation: An overview. Nurs Forum 1974;13:240-258.

Bond M: Assessment of the psychosocial outcome of severe head injury. In outcome of severe damage to the central nervous system. Ciba Foundation Symposium. Elsevier, Amsterdam, 1975;34:141-143.

Bond MR: Assessment of the psychological outcome after severe head injury. Acta Neurochir (Wein) 1976;34:57.

Brickett F, Pigott R: Visual neglect. Am J Nurs 1966;66:101-105.

Bricolo A, Turazzi S, Feriotto G: Prolonged post-traumatic unconsciousness: Therapeutic assets and liabilities. J Neurosurg 1980;52:625.

Brink J, Imbus C, Woo-Sam J: Physical recovery after severe closed head trauma in children and adults. J Pediatr 1980;97: 721-727.

Brooks DN, Aughton ME: Psychological consequences of blunt head injury. Rehabilitation Medicine 1979;1(4):160-165.

Bruce D, Schut L, Raphaeley RE, et al: Outcome following severe head injury in children. J Neurosurg 1978;489:679-688.

Carlson CA, von Essen C, Lofgren J: Factors affecting clinical course of patients with severe head injuries. J Neurosurg 1968;29:242.

Carlssen CA, Von Essen C, Logfren J: Factors affecting the clinical course of patients with severe head trauma. Part 1: influence of biological factors. Part 2: Significance of post-traumatic coma. J Neurosurg 1968;29:242.

Chusid J, McDonald J: Correlative Neuroanatomy and Functional Neurology. Lange Medical Publications, Los Altos, Calif, 1967.

Cope DN, Hall K: Head injury rehabilitation: Benefit of early intervention. Arch Phys Med Rehabil 1982;63:433.

Darley FL, Aronson AE, Brown JR: Motor Speech Disorders. WB Saunders Co, Philadelphia, 1975.

DeMeyer W: Technique of the Neurologic Examination. McGraw-Hill Book Co, New York, 1974.

DeRenzi E, Vignolo LA: The token test: A sensitive test to detect receptive disturbances in aphasics. Brain 1962;85:665.

Diller L, Gordon W: Interventions for cognitive deficits in brain injured adults. J Consult Clin Psychol 1981;49:822-834.

Diller L: A model for cognitive retraining in rehabilitation. Clinical Psychologist 1976;6:13.

Dimkens MA, Temkin N: Neuropsychologic outcome at one month post injury. Arch Phys Med Rehabil 1986;67:507.

Dinsdale S, et al: Problem oriented medical records: Their impact on staff communication. Arch Phys Med Rehabil 1975;56:269.

DiSimoni FG: Assessment factors in effective treatment of aphasic patients. Journal of Pennsylvania Speech and Hearing Association 1980;8:2.

Eiben CF, Anderson TP, Lockman L, et al: Functional outcome of closed head injury in children and young adults. Arch Phys Med Rehabil 1984,65:168-170.

Fiorentino MR: Reflex Testing Methods for Evaluating Central Nervous System Development. Ed 2. Charles C Thomas Publisher, Springfield, Ill, 1973.

Fischer RP, Carlson J, Perry JD: Postconcussive hospital observation of alert patients in primary trauma center. J Trauma 1981;21(11):920-924.

Fodor IE: Impairment of memory functions after acute head injury. J Neurol Neurosurg Psychiatry 1972;35:818-824.

Friedlander WT: Anosognosia and perception. Am J Phys Med 1967;46:1394-1408.

Fuld PA, Fisher P: Recovery of intellectual ability after closed head injury. Dev Med Child Neurol 1977;19:495-502.

Galbraith S, Murray WR, Pater AR, et al: The relationship between alcohol and head injury and its effects on the conscious level. Br J Surg 1976;63:128.

Gilchrist E, Wilkinson M: Some factors determining prognosis in young people with severe head injuries. Arch Neurol 1979;36;355-359.

Gjone R, Kristiansen K, Sponheim N: Rehabilitation in severe head injuries. Scand J Rehabil Med 1972;4:2-4.

Graham DI, Adams JH, Doyle D: Ischaemic brain damage in fatal non-missile head injuries. J Neurol Sci 1978;39:213.

Granger CV, Delabarre EM Jr: Programmed examination formats: Use in rehabilitation medicine. Arch Phys Med Rehabil 1974;55:235.

Groher M: Language and memory disorders following closed head trauma. J Speech Hear Res 1977;20:212.

Gronwall D, Wrightson P: Memory and information processing capacity after closed head injury. J Neurol Neurosurg Psychiatry 1981;44(10):889-895.

Haberman B: Cognitive dysfunction and social rehabilitation in the severely head injured patient. Journal of Neurosurgery-Nursing 1982;14(5):220-224.

Hagen C: Language disorders secondary to closed head injury: Diagnosis and treatment. Topics in Language Disorders 1981;1:73-87.

Hannay HJ, Levin HS, Grossman RG: Impaired recognition memory after head injury. Cortex 1979;15(2):269-283.

Heiskanen O, Sipponen P: Prognosis of severe brain injury. Acta Neurol Scand 1970;46:343.

Hilson A: The physiology of spasticity. Postgrad Med J 1972;4B:25-27.

Jeannett B: Some aspects of prognosis after severe head injury. Scand J Rehabil Med 1972;4:16-20.

Jeannett B, Bond M: Assessment of outcome after severe brain damage. Lancet 1975;1:480-484.

Jeannett B: Prognosis after severe head injury. Clin Neurosurg 1972;19:200.

Jeannett B: Prognosis of patients with severe head injury. Neurosurgery 1979;4(4):283.

Jeannett B: Predicting outcome in individual patients after severe head injury. Lancet 1976;1:1031.

Kishore PRS, et al: Delayed development of hydrocephalus in patients with severe head injury. Neuroradiology 1978;16:261.

Knott M, Voss D: Proprioceptive Neuromuscular Facilitation. Ed 2. Harper & Row Publishers Inc, New York, 1968.

Kornhubers HH (Ed): The Somatosensory System. Ed 3. Publishing Sciences Group, 1975.

Levati A, Farina ML, Vecchi G, et al: Prognosis of severe head injuries. J Neurosurg 1982;57(6):779-783.

Levin H, Benton A, Grossman R: Neurobehavioral Consequences of Closed Head Injury. Oxford University Press Inc, New York, 1982.

Levin HS, Grossman RG, Sarwar M, et al: Linguistic recovery after closed head injury. Brain Lang 1981;12(2):360-374.

Lewinn EB: The coma arousal team. R Soc Health 1980;10:19.

Lobato RD, Cordobes F, Rivas JS, et al: Outcome from severe head injury related to the type of intracranial lesion: A computerized tomography study. J Neurosurg 1983;59:767-774.

Malec J, Questad K: Rehabilitation of memory after craniocerebral trauma case report. Arch Phys Med Rehabil 1983;64:436.

Mandelburg IA: Cognitive recovery after severe head injury. Wechsler Adult Intelligence Scale during post-traumatic anmesia. J Neurol Neurosurg Psychiatry 1975;38:1127.

Marshall LF, Smith RW, Shapiro HM: The outcome with aggressive treatment in severe head injuries. J Neurosurg 1979;50:26.

McGraw MB: The Neuromuscular Maturation of the Human Infant. Hafner Press, NY, 1945.

Meichenbaum D: Cognitive behavior modification: An integrative approach. Plenum Press, New York, 1977.

Melvin JL: Interdisciplinary and multidisciplinary activities. Arch Phys Med Rehabil 1980;61:379.

Miller JD, Sweet RC, Narayon R, et al: Early insults to the injured brain. JAMA 1978;240:439.

Milhous RL: Problem oriented medical record in rehabilitation management and training. Arch Phys Med Rehabil 1970;53:488.

Milner B: Residual intellectual and memory deficits after head injury. In Walker AE (Ed): The Late Effects of Head Injury. Charles C Thomas Publisher, Springfield, Ill, 1969.

Molner GE (Ed): Pediatric Rehabilitation. Williams & Wilkins Co, Baltimore, 1985.

Overgaard J, Hansen D, Land AM, et al: Prognosis after head injury based on early clinical evaluation. Lancet 1973;2:631.

Pazzaglia P, et al: Clinical course and prognosis of acute post-traumatic coma. J Neurol Neurosurg Psychiatry 1975;38:149.

Peterson GC: Organic brain syndromes associated with brain trauma. In Freedman AM, et al: Comprehensive Textbook of Psychiatry. Williams & Wilkins Co, Baltimore, 1975, pp 1093-1108.

Reinstein L, Staas W, Marquette C: A rehabilitation evaluation system which compliments the problem oriented medical record. Arch Phys Med Rehabil 1975;56:396.

Rimel RW, Giordani B, Barth JT, et al: Moderate head injury: Completing the clinical spectrum of brain trauma. Neurosurgery 1982;11(3):344-351.

Romano M: Family response to traumatic head injury. Scand J Rehabil Med 1974;6:1-4.

Rood MS: Neurophysiological mechanisms utilized in treatment of neuromuscular dysfunction. Am J Occup Ther 1956;10(4):220-224.

Russell WR, Smith A: Post traumatic anmesia in closed head injury. Arch Neurol 1961;5:4.

Sandel ME, Abrams PL, Horn LJ: Hypertension after brain injury: Case report. Arch Phys Med Rehabil 1986;67:469.

Sarno MT: The nature of verbal impairment after closed head injury. J Nerv Ment Dis. 1980;168(11):685-692.

Seales DM, Rossiter VS, Weinstein ME: Brainstem auditory evoked responses in patients comatose as a result of blunt head trauma. J Trauma 1979;19(5):347-353.

Smith RM: Prognosis after severe head trauma, Fourth Annual Post-Graduate Course on the Rehabilitation of the Traumatic Brain Injured Adult. Williamsburg, Va, 1980.

Smith RM, et al: A functional scale of recovery from severe head trauma. Clin Neuropsychol 1979;1:48.

Smith RM: Prognosis of aphasia: Etiology, time and linguistic factors. Proceedings of the International Association of Logopedics, Washington, DC, 1981.

Springer SP, Deutsch G: Left Brain, Right Brain. WH Freeman and Co, San Francisco, 1981.

Stablein DM, et al: Statistical methods for determining prognosis in severe head injury. Neurosurgery 1980;6:243.

Switzer D: Dynamics of Grief. Abingdon Press, NY, 1970.

Symonds CP: Concussion and its sequellae. Lancet 1962;1:1.

Teasdale G, Jeannett B: Assessment of coma and impaired consciousness: A practical scale. Lancet 1974;2:81-84.

Urosevich P, Obenrader M, Graham N: Providing for early mobility. Intermed Communications Inc, Horsham, Penn, 1980. Vapalahti M, Troupp H: Prognosis for patients with severe brain injuries. Br Med J 1971;3:404.

Verbanets J (Ed): Head Injury: Topics in Acute Care and Trauma Rehabilitation. Vol 1, No 1. Aspen Publishers Inc, Rockville, Md, July 1986. Walker AE: Long term evaluation of the social and family adjustment to head injuries. Scand J Rehabil Med 1972;4:5-8.

Wallhagen MI: The split brain: Implications for care and rehabilitation. Am J Nurs 1979;79(12):2118-2125.

Weber PL: Sensorimotor therapy: Its effects on EEGs of acute combat patients. Arch Phys Med Rehabil 1984;65:457.

Yarkony G, et al: Rehabilitation of craniocerebral trauma. Ann Acad Med Singapore 1983;12:417-421.

Zimmerman RA, et al: Computed tomography of pediatric head trauma: Acute general cerebral swelling. Radiology 1978;126:403.

APPENDIX A
PHYSICAL THERAPY HISTORY/ CARE PLAN

PHYSICAL THERAPY EVALUATION

PATIENT: _____ AGE: _____
DATE OF ONSET: _____
DATE(S) OF EVALUATION: _____

I.   HISTORY: Primary Injury/Type: _____

Location: _____
Mechanism: _____
Secondary Injuries (Type, location, weight bearing status:)
_____

Surgical interventions/dates: _____

Initial responses (GCS Score)/changes: _____

Premorbid medical/social history (handedness, support
systems): _____

Current medications/route/dosage: _____

Pertinent test results (evoked potentials, EMG, x-ray, CT
scans, etc.): _____
_____

II. GENERAL OBSERVATIONS: (Status without interaction, e.g.,
     posturing, spontaneous movement, response to environment,
     agitation)

III. TEST RESULTS

IV. CURRENT FINDINGS/ASSESSMENT: Cognitive Level _____
     (Summary of abilities and limitations, major problems,
     areas amenable to therapeutic intervention)

V.   PLAN: Goals, treatment plan

APPENDIX B
COGNITIVE/BEHAVIORAL
ASSESSMENT

COGNITIVE/BEHAVIORAL ASSESSMENT

	NEVER	50% OF TIME	50-75% TIME	75-100% TIME	COMMENTS
Responds to pain					
Generalized response to stimulation					
Localized response to stimulation					
Delayed response to stimulation					
Focuses					
Tracks					
Oriented to person					
Oriented to place					
Oriented to time					
Remembers therapist's name (during session)					
Remembers therapist's name (from session to session)					
Responds yes/no					
Initiates conversation					
Initiates activity					
Follows commands - 1 step					
Follows commands - 2 steps					
Follows commands - 3 steps					
Agitated					
Confused					
Impulsive					
Irritable					
Distractable					
Impersistent					
Perseverative					
Combative					
Lethargic					
Anxious					

APPENDIX C
MUSCULOSKELETAL ASSESSMENT

PHYSICAL THERAPY ASSESSMENT

PROM	TONE	MOTOR	COMMENTS		PROM	TONE	MOTOR	COMMENTS
				NECK:				
				Flexion				
				Extension				
				Lateral flexion				
				Rotation				
				TRUNK:				
				Flexion				
				Extension				
				Lateral flexion				
				Rotation				
				HIP:				
				Flexion				
				Straight leg raise				
				Extension				
				Abduction				
				Adduction				
				Internal rotation				
				External rotation				
				KNEE:				
				Flexion				
				Extension				
				ANKLE:				
				Dorsiflexion				
				Plantarflexion				
				Eversion				
				Inversion				
				TOES:				
				Flexion				
				Extension				
				Abduction				
				SCAPULA:				
				Elevation				
				Depression				
				Protraction				
				Retraction				

MUSCULOSKELETAL ASSESSMENT
CONTINUED

PHYSICAL THERAPY ASSESSMENT

COMMENTS	MOTOR	TONE	PROM		PROM	TONE	MOTOR	COMMENTS
				SHOULDER:				
				Flexion				
				Extension				
				Abduction				
				Adduction				
				Horizontal abduction				
				Horizontal adduction				
				Internal rotation				
				External rotation				
				ELBOW:				
				Flexion				
				Extension				
				FOREARM:				
				Supination				
				Pronation				
				WRIST:				
				Flexion				
				Extension				
				Radial deviation				
				Ulnar deviation				
				FINGERS:				
				Metacarpal flexion				
				Metacarpal extension				
				Interphalangeal flexion				
				Interphalangeal extension				
				Abduction				
				Adduction				
				THUMB:				
				Metacarpal flexion				
				Metacarpal extension				
				Interphalangeal flexion				
				Interphalangeal extension				
				Abduction				
				Adduction				
				Opposition				
				GRASP:				
				Pinch				

MUSCULOSKELETAL ASSESSMENT
CONTINUED

PHYSICAL THERAPY ASSESSMENT

COMMENTS	MOTOR	TONE	PROM		PROM	TONE	MOTOR	COMMENTS
				GRASP (Continued): Lateral pinch Three jaw chuck Hook Large grasp				

APPENDIX D
SENSORY EVALUATION

			LEFT			RIGHT			
LE	UE	TRUNK	FACE	SENSATION	FACE	TRUNK	UE	LE
				Pain				
				Temperature				
				Sharp/dull				
				Pressure				
				Light touch				
				Localization				
				Extinctions				
				Proprioception				
				Kinesthesia				

COMMENTS:

KEY: + = Intact
− = Absent
± = Impaired

APPENDIX E
REFLEX ASSESSMENT

PHYSICAL THERAPY ASSESSMENT

LUE	LLE	REFLEXES	RUE	RLE
		Spinal level: Flexor withdrawal Extensor thurst Crossed extension - flexion Crossed extension - extension		

		Brainstem level:
		Asymmetrical tonic neck reflex
		  Neck rotation to right
		  Neck rotation to left
		Symmetrical tonic neck reflex
		  Flexion
		  Extension
		Asymmetrical tonic labyrinthine reflex
		  Right sidelying
		  Left sidelying
		Symmetrical tonic labyrinthine reflex
		  Supine
		  Prone
		Positive supporting reaction
		Negative supporting reaction		

		Midbrain:
		Neck righting
		Body righting
		Labyrinthine righting
		  Prone
		  Supine
		  Right sidelying
		  Left sidelying
		Optical righting
		  Prone
		  Supine
		  Right sidelying
		  Left sidelying		

		Cortical:
		Equilibrium reactions
		Supine
		  Displace to right
		  Displace to left
		Sitting
		  Displace anteriorally
		  Displace posteriorally
		  Displace laterally to right
		  Displace laterally to left
		Standing
		  Displace anteriorally
		  Displace posteriorally
		  Displace laterally to right
		  Displace laterally to left		

KEY: + = Present   - = Absent   ± = Variable

APPENDIX F
GROSS MOTOR CONTROL

CHART V: Gross Motor Control

KEY: + = Intact
    – = Absent
    +/– = Developing

POSTURE:	MOBILITY — Able to be positioned	MOBILITY — Assists to position	STABILITY — Maintains position	CONTROLLED MOBILITY — Assumes position	CONTROLLED MOBILITY — Weight shifts	CONTROLLED MOBILITY — Segmentally rotates	STATIC- — Counter-rotates	STATIC- — Lifts one point of support	STATIC- — Lifts two points of support	SKILL — Lifts two points of support	SKILL — Locomotes	COMMENTS
Initial upright progression:												
Right sidelying												
Left sidelying												
Sitting												
Prone progression:												
Prone on elbows												
Quadruped												
Lower trunk progression:												
Lower trunk rotation												
Bridging												
Kneeling												
Half-kneeling												
Advanced upright progression:												
Modified plantigrade												
Standing												
OTHER:												

APPENDIX G
BALANCE ASSESSMENT

EVALUATION OF BALANCE	Unable	Maintains	Against resistance	Accepts challenge	COMMENTS
SITTING:					
With bilateral upper extremity support					
With unilateral upper extremity support					
Without support					
STANDING: Basic stance with bilateral upper extremity support					
With unilateral upper extremity support					
Without support					
Unilateral stance: Right: with bilateral upper extremity support					
Right: with unilateral upper extremity support					
Right: without support					
Left: with bilateral upper extremity support					
Left: with unilateral upper extremity support					
Left: without support					

SKIN CONDITION: (Descriptive)

RESPIRATORY STATUS: (Descriptive)

APPENDIX H
MOVEMENT DISORDERS

	HEAD	TRUNK	RUE	LUE	LLE	LUE	COMMENTS
Ataxia - dysynergia Ataxia - dysmetria							
Tremor							
Dystonia							
Athetoid movements							
Ballismic movements							
Choreiform movements							
Dysdiadochokinesia							
Bradykinesia							

KEY: + = Marked
     - = None
     $\pm$ = Mild

APPENDIX I
FUNCTIONAL ABILITIES

Functional Abilities

ACTIVITY	UNABLE	WITH ASSIST	WITH CUES	INDEPENDENT	COMMENTS
BED MOBILITY:					
1. Vertical					
2. Horizontal					
3. Rolling					
4. Supine (edge of bed sitting)					
TRANSFERS:					
Bed					
Wheelchair					
Toilet					
Car					
Floor					
WHEELCHAIR MOBILITY:					
Preparation					
Level					
Uneven					
Ramps					
Doors					
Elevators					
AMBULATORY STATUS:					
Preparation					
Level					
Uneven					
Doors					
Stairs					

APPENDIX J
POSTURAL ANALYSIS

POSTURE	SUPINE		SITTING		STANDING	
	L	R	L	R	L	R
HEAD:						
Midline						
Lordosis						
Flexion						
Extension						
Protraction						
Rotation						
Lateral flexion						
SCAPULA:						
Symmetrical						
Elevation						
Depression						
Protraction						
Retraction						
Upward rotation						
Downward rotation						
TRUNK:						
Symmetrical						
Rotation						
Lateral flexion						
Flexion						
Extension						
Kyphosis						
PELVIS:						
Symmetrical						
Anterior tilt						
Posterior tilt						
Protraction						
Retraction						
UPPER EXTREMITIES:						
Symmetrical						
Flexion - Shoulder						
Extension - Shoulder						
Abduction - Shoulder						
Adduction - Shoulder						
Internal Rotation						
External Rotation						
Shoulder						
Elbow						
Forearm						
Supination						
Pronation						
Wrist flexion						
Wrist extension						
Radial deviation						
Ulnar deviation						
Finger flexion						
Finger extension						
Finger abduction						
Finger adduction						

KEY: + = Present   - = Not present

POSTURAL ANALYSIS
CONTINUED

POSTURE	SUPINE		SITTING		STANDING	
	L	R	L	R	L	R
UPPER EXTREMITIES (Continued):						
Thumb abduction						
Thumb adduction						
LOWER EXTREMITIES:						
Hip flexion						
Hip extension						
Hip abduction						
Hip adduction						
Hip internal rotation						
Hip external rotation						
Knee flexion						
Knee extension						
Ankle plantarflexion						
Ankle inversion						
Toe flexion						

KEY: + = Present   - = Not Present

APPENDIX K
GAIT ANALYSIS

STANCE		TRUNK	SWING	
L	R		L	R
		Forward		
		Backward		
		Lordosis		
		Rotation		
		Lateral bend		
		PELVIS:		
		Retraction		
		Protraction		
		Hike		
		Anterior tilt		
		Posterior tilt		
		Trendelenburg		
		SHOULDER GIRDLE:		
		Retraction		
		Protraction		
		Elevation		
		Reciprocal arm swing		
		HIP:		
		Excessive flexion		
		Inadequate flexion		
		Circumduction		
		Adduction		
		Abduction		
		Internal rotation		
		External rotation		
		KNEE:		
		Hyperextension		
		Excessive flexion		
		Insufficient flexion		
		Buckling		
		ANKLE:		
		Heel contact		
		Inversion		
		Excessive dorsiflexion		
		Inadequate dorsiflesion		
		Unstable		
		TOES:		
		Extended		
		Clawing		
		Pronation		
		Supination		
		COMMENTS: Weight bearing status, BOS, cadence, step length, weight shift, distance, orthotic device, assistive devise, assistance required, description of upper extremity posturing.		

APPENDIX L
EVALUATION FOR POST ACUTE REHABILITATION (LOW LEVEL PATIENT)

EVALUATION FOR POST ACUTE REHABILITATION
(Low Level Patient)

AGE: _____   DATE OF ONSET: _____

DIAGNOSIS (Head Injury): _____

DIAGNOSIS (Other Injuries): _____
_____

Initial Glasgow Score: _____   Cognitive Level_____

I. LEVEL OF AWARENESS:
A. Present Glasgow Score: _____
B. Rancho Los Amigos Cognitive Level: _____
C. Response to Command: Immediate ___ Delayed ___ None ___
D. Medication/Route:_____
_____

  Sedatives: _____
  Anticonvulsant(s): _____
E. History of hydrocephalus: _____ Yes _____ No
F. Shunt performed: _____ Yes (give date) _____ No

II. MEDICAL STABILITY:
A. Cardiovascular:
  1. Blood pressure: _____
  2. History of hypertension: _____ Yes _____ No
  3. Pulse: _____
  4. History of cardiac or vascular problems: ___ Yes ___ No
B. Respiratory:
  1. Pneumothorax: _____
  2. Mechanical ventilation: _____
  3. Tracheostomy: (describe secretions/give date of surgery)
_____
  4. Pneumonia: _____
  5. CPT: _____
  6. Oxygen: _____
C. Seizures:
  1. History of seizure activity: _____
_____
  2. Date of most recent seizure: _____
  3. Date of prior seizure(s): _____

LOW LEVEL PATIENT
CONTINUED

C. Seizures (Continued):

    4. Medication(s)/dosage: _____

    5. Last serum level: _____
    6. Description of seizure activity: _____
    _____

D. Infection:

    1. Most recent tracheostomy C&S: _____
    2. Most recent gastrostomy C&S: _____
    3. Most recent urine C&S: _____
    4. Most recent wound C&S: _____
    5. History of infection: _____

    6. Present antibiotics: _____

    7. Present febrile episodes: _____
    _____

E. Skin:

    1. History of decubiti: _____
    2. Present skin condition: _____
    3. Treatment(s): _____
    _____

III. **PHYSICAL ABILITY IMPAIRMENTS (Check all that apply):**

A. _____ Fractures (describe below)
B. _____ Contractures (describe below)
C. _____ Spasticity
D. _____ Flaccidity
E. _____ Decreased endurance
F. _____ Heterotopic Ossification (describe below)
G. _____ Movement pattern/reflexive level (describe below)

COMMENTS: _____
_____
_____
_____
_____

LOW LEVEL PATIENT
CONTINUED

IV. SENSORY FUNCTION/IMPAIRMENT:

		Intact	Delayed	Absent
A.	Tactile	___	___	___
B.	Auditory	___	___	___
C.	Visual	___	___	___
D.	Olfactory	___	___	___

COMMENTS: _____
_____
_____

V. PERCEPTUAL FUNCTION/IMPAIRMENT:

		Consistent	Inconsistent	Absent
A.	Focusing	___	___	___
B.	Tracking	___	___	___
C.	Crossing Midline:			
	Visual	___	___	___
	Motor	___	___	___

COMMENTS: _____
_____
_____

VI. DIAGNOSTIC STUDIES:

A. Initial CT scan date/results: _____

B. Latest CT scan date/result: _____

C. Evoked potential date/results: _____

Therapy involvement to date: _____
_____
_____

APPENDIX M
EVALUATION FOR POST ACUTE
REHABILITATION (AGITATED
PATIENT)

EVALUATION FOR POST ACUTE REHABILITATION
(Agitated Patient)

AGE: _____   DATE OF ONSET: _____

DIAGNOSIS: _____
_____
_____

INITIAL GLASGOW COMA SCORE: _____

MEDICATION/ROUTE: _____
_____
_____

MEDICAL PROBLEMS:

	Severe	Moderate	None
Seizures:			
Controlled	____	____	____
Uncontrolled	____	____	____
Hypertension	____	____	____
Tracheostomy	____	____	____
Gastrostomy	____	____	____
Decubiti	____	____	____
Infectious	____	____	____

COMMENTS: _____
_____
_____

PHYSICAL IMPAIRMENTS/MOTOR FUNCTION PROBLEMS:

	Severe	Moderate	None
Fractures	____	____	____
Contractures	____	____	____
Spasticity	____	____	____
Decreased endurance	____	____	____
Heterotopic ossification	____	____	____
Impaired ambulation	____	____	____
Impaired w/c mobility	____	____	____
Impaired positioning	____	____	____
Impaired transfer ability	____	____	____

AGITATED PATIENT
CONTINUED

	Severe	Moderate	None
Impaired fine motor coordination	_____	_____	_____
Impaired gross motor coordination	_____	_____	_____
Speech Production	_____	_____	_____

COMMENTS: _____
_____
_____

COGNITIVE IMPAIRMENTS:

	Severe	Moderate	None
Impaired Memory	_____	_____	_____
Confusion	_____	_____	_____
Disorientation	_____	_____	_____
Delayed Processing	_____	_____	_____
Impaired verbal comprehension	_____	_____	_____
Impaired word finding	_____	_____	_____
Delayed response	_____	_____	_____
Verbal excitement	_____	_____	_____

COMMENTS: _____
_____
_____

BEHAVIORAL PROBLEMS:

	Severe	Moderate	None
Restlessness	_____	_____	_____
Impaired impulse control	_____	_____	_____
Verbal abusiveness	_____	_____	_____
Physical aggression (predictable)	_____	_____	_____
Physical aggression (unpredictable)	_____	_____	_____
Wandering	_____	_____	_____

COMMENTS: _____
_____
_____

Physical Restraints Used: _____ Yes   _____ No

AGITATED PATIENT
CONTINUED

Length of agitated state to date: _____
Number of outbursts daily: _____
Usual duration of outbursts: _____
Precipitating factors: _____
_____
_____
_____

History of therapy involvement: _____
_____
_____
_____
_____

APPENDIX N
FUNCTIONAL ASSESSMENT
(MID TO HIGH LEVEL PATIENT)

FUNCTIONAL ASSESSMENT
Mid to High Level Patient

AGE: _____   DATE OF ONSET: _____

DATE OF EVALUATION: _____

COGNITIVE LEVEL: _____

PRESENT MEDICATION(S)/DOSAGE/ROUTE: _____
_____
_____

MEDICAL PROBLEMS: (If yes is checked, describe in comments):

	YES	NO
Cardiac	_____	_____
Respiratory	_____	_____
Infectious	_____	_____
Fractures	_____	_____
Decubiti	_____	_____
Hypertension	_____	_____
Tracheostomy	_____	_____
Gastrostomy	_____	_____
Nasogastric Tube	_____	_____
Bladder Continence	_____	_____
Bowel Continence	_____	_____
Shunt	_____	_____
Seizures (and date most recent)	_____ Date: _____	_____

COMMENTS: _____
_____
_____
_____
_____

MID TO HIGH LEVEL PATIENT
CONTINUED

MOTOR FUNCTION:

	No Impairment	Mild	Moderate	Severe
Strength:				
RUE	_____	_____	_____	_____
LUE	_____	_____	_____	_____
RLE	_____	_____	_____	_____
LLE	_____	_____	_____	_____
Range of Motion:				
RUE	_____	_____	_____	_____
LUE	_____	_____	_____	_____
RLE	_____	_____	_____	_____
LLE	_____	_____	_____	_____
Endurance	_____	_____	_____	_____
Muscle tone	_____	_____	_____	_____
Gross Motor control	_____	_____	_____	_____
Fine Motor control	_____	_____	_____	_____
Oral/Motor	_____	_____	_____	_____

	Independent	W/Assist	Unable
Balance	_____	_____	_____
Transfers	_____	_____	_____
Ambulation	_____	_____	_____

SENSORY/SENSORY—MOTOR FUNCTION:

	Intact	Impaired	Absent
Vision (track/focus)	_____	_____	_____
Auditory discrimination	_____	_____	_____
Tactile discrimination	_____	_____	_____
Right/left discrimination	_____	_____	_____
Body part awareness	_____	_____	_____
Bilateral motor integration	_____	_____	_____
Motor planning	_____	_____	_____

PERCEPTUAL FUNCTION:

	Intact	Impaired	Absent
Ability to cross midline	_____	_____	_____
Figure ground discrimination	_____	_____	_____
Position in space	_____	_____	_____
Depth perception	_____	_____	_____
Spatial relations	_____	_____	_____
Visual/motor integration	_____	_____	_____

MID TO HIGH LEVEL PATIENT
CONTINUED

ACTIVITIES OF DAILY LIVING:

	Independent	W/Assist	Unable
Bathing	____	____	____
Dressing	____	____	____
Toileting	____	____	____
Self-feeding	____	____	____
Grooming	____	____	____

COGNITIVE FUNCTION:

	Intact	Impaired	Absent
Memory:			
Long term	____	____	____
Short term	____	____	____
Immediate	____	____	____
Language skills (receptive):			
Reading comprehension	____	____	____
Auditory comprehension	____	____	____
Auditory discrimination	____	____	____
Word recognition	____	____	____
Language skills (expressive):			
Verbal expression	____	____	____
Word finding	____	____	____
Fluency	____	____	____
Gestural communication	____	____	____
Orientation:			
Person	____	____	____
Place	____	____	____
Time	____	____	____
Attention	____	____	____
Problem Solving	____	____	____
Decision Making	____	____	____
Judgment	____	____	____
Sequencing	____	____	____
Insight	____	____	____
Behavior/Social/ Psychological:			
Impulse Control	____	____	____
Emotional Stability	____	____	____
Interpersonal Skills	____	____	____
Self Control	____	____	____
Initiative	____	____	____
Frustration Tolerance	____	____	____
Coping Skills	____	____	____

MID TO HIGH LEVEL PATIENT
CONTINUED

COMMENTS: _____

_____

_____

OTHER PSYCHOLOGICAL/BEHAVIORAL PROBLEMS (check all that apply):

Decreased self-esteem   _____
Impaired motivation   _____
Depression   _____
Anxiety   _____
Impaired assertiveness   _____
Verbally abusive   _____
Physically aggressive   _____
Sexual problems   _____
Over-dependency   _____
Inappropriate affect   _____
Suicidal ideation   _____
Acting out   _____

SPEECH FUNCTION:

	Yes	No
Verbal communicator	_____	_____
Dysarthria	_____	_____
Oral/motor apraxia	_____	_____
*Non-verbal communicator	_____	_____

*If yes, indicate the type of communication system utilized:

_____
_____
_____

25.35